Charting

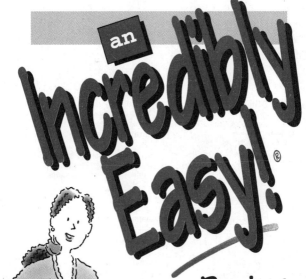

an **Incredibly Easy!**®

Pocket
Guide

‖‖‖‖‖‖‖‖‖‖‖‖‖‖‖‖‖‖‖‖‖‖‖‖‖‖
W9-COE-135

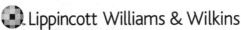

Lippincott Williams & Wilkins
a Wolters Kluwer business
Philadelphia · Baltimore · New York · London
Buenos Aires · Hong Kong · Sydney · Tokyo

Staff

Executive Publisher
Judith A. Schilling McCann, RN, MSN

Editorial Director
David Moreau

Clinical Director
Joan M. Robinson, RN, MSN

Art Director
Mary Ludwicki

Senior Managing Editor
Jaime Stockslager Buss, ELS

Clinical Manager
Collette Bishop Hendler, RN, BS, CCRN

Clinical Project Manager
Cynthia Brophy, RN, BSN, CPAN

Editors
Liz Schaeffer, Gale Thompson,
Beth Wegerbauer

Clinical Editor
Marcy Caplin, RN, MSN

Copy Editors
Kimberly Bilotta (supervisor),
Jane Bradford, Lisa Stockslager,
Dorothy P. Terry, Pamela Wingrod

Designer
Lynn Foulk

Illustrator
Bot Roda

Digital Composition Services
Diane Paluba (manager), Joyce Rossi Biletz,
Donna S. Morris

Associate Manufacturing Manager
Beth J. Welsh

Editorial Assistants
Megan L. Aldinger, Karen J. Kirk,
Linda K. Ruhf

Design Assistant
Georg W. Purvis IV

Indexer
Barbara Hodgson

CHIEPG011106—020607

Library of Congress Cataloging-in-Publication Data
Charting : an incredibly easy pocket guide.
    p. ; cm.
    Includes bibliographical references and index.
    1. Nursing records—Handbooks, manuals,
    etc. I. Lippincott Williams & Wilkins.
    [DNLM: 1. Nursing Records—Handbooks. 2.
    Documentation—Handbooks.
    WY 49 C486 2007]
RT50.C4433 2007
610.73—dc22
ISBN-13: 978-1-58255-538-6
ISBN-10: 1-58255-538-9 (alk. paper)   2006025286

Contents

Contributors and consultants iv

Road map to charting v

A–C 1
D–H 81
I–N 153
O–Q 213
R–Z 295

Appendices and index

The test zone 373
JCAHO National Patient Safety Goals 386
Electronic health record 392
Selected references 397
Index 399

Contributors and consultants

Adrianne E. Avillion, RN, DEd
President
AEA Consulting
York, Pa.

Peggy Bozarth, RN, MSN
Professor
Hopkinsville (Ky.) Community College

Cheryl L. Brady, RN, MSN
Nurse Educator
Youngstown (Ohio) State University

Virginia L. Branson, RN, MA, CBCS
Program Director — Medical Office
   Management
Virginia College
Birmingham, Ala.

Christine Greenidge, RN, MSN, BC
Director of Nursing Professional Practice
Montefiore Medical Center
Bronx, N.Y.

Merita Konstantacos, RN, MSN
Consultant
Clinton, Ohio

Theresa Pulvano, RN, BSN
Nursing Educator
Ocean County Vocational Technical School,
   Practical Nursing Program
Lakehurst, N.J.

Roseanne Hanlon Rafter, APRN,BC, MSN
Director of Nursing Professional Practice
Pottstown (Pa.) Memorial Medical Center

Elsa Nicklas Sanchez, RN, BSN, BA
Staff Development
Meadowview Nursing Home Atlantic
   County
Northfield, N.J.

Rita M. Wick, RN, BSN
Education Specialist
Berkshire Health Systems
Pittsfield, Mass.

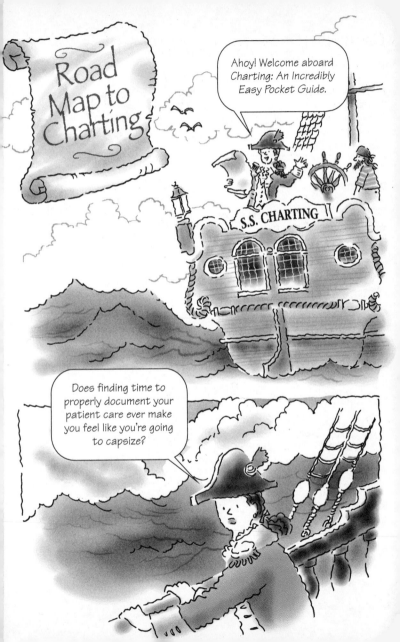

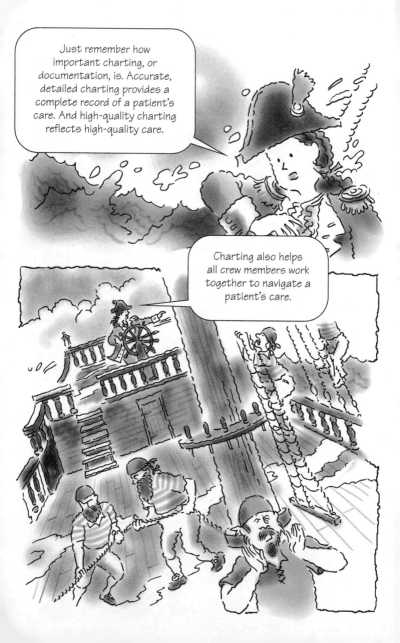

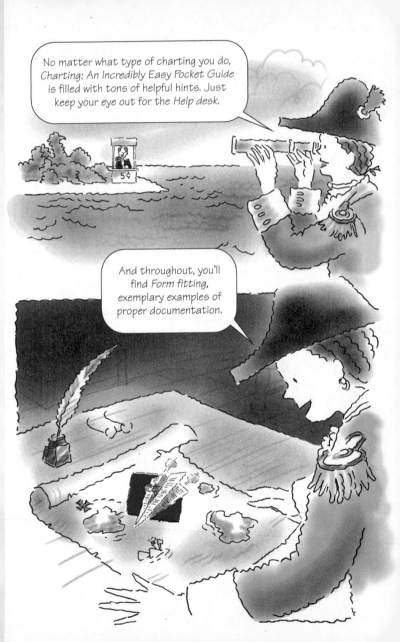

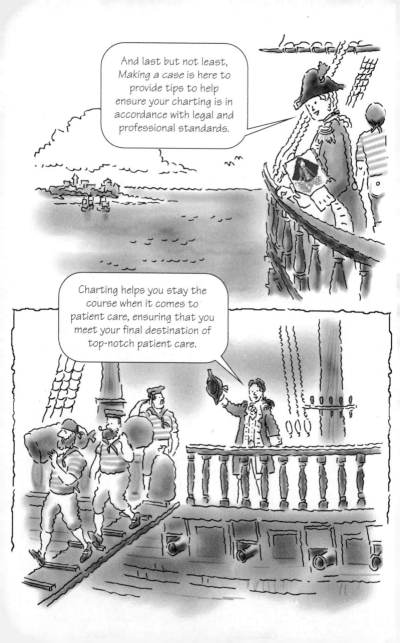

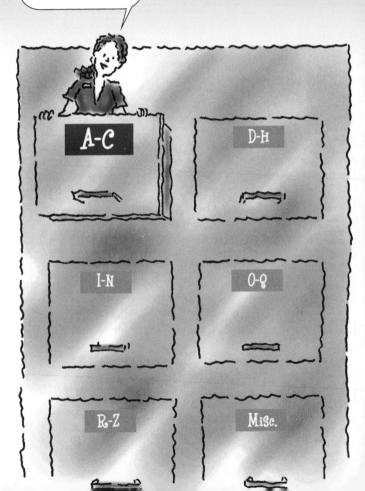
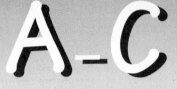

A

Abuse suspicions

- Abuse may occur in any age-group, cultural setting, or environment.
- The patient may readily report abuse or fear reporting the abuser.
- Types of abuse include:
  - neglect
  - physical abuse
  - sexual abuse
  - emotional abuse
  - psychological abuse.
- In most states, a nurse is required by law to report signs of abuse in children, the elderly, and the disabled.
- Report your suspicions to the appropriate administrator and agency.
- Document suspicions on the appropriate form or in your nurse's notes.
- If the victim's caregiver is present, interview the victim and the caregiver separately to note inconsistencies with histories.
- An injunction can be obtained to separate the abuser and the abused until circumstances can be investigated.
- Certain cultural practices, such as coin rubbing in Vietnamese cultures, produce bruises or burns that may be mistaken for abuse.
- The final judgment of child abuse is decided by social services and the health care team.

Common signs of neglect and abuse

Neglect
- Failure to thrive in infants
- Malnutrition
- Dehydration
- Poor personal hygiene
- Inadequate clothing
- Severe diaper rash
- Injuries from falls
- Failure of wounds to heal
- Periodontal disease
- Infestations, such as scabies, lice, or maggots in a wound

Abuse
- Recurrent injuries
- Multiple injuries or fractures in various stages of healing
- Unexplained bruises, abrasions, burns, bites, damaged or missing teeth, strap or rope marks
- Head injuries or bald spots from pulling out hair
- Bleeding from body orifices
- Genital trauma
- Sexually transmitted diseases in children
- Pregnancy in young girls or women with physical or mental handicaps
- Verbalized accounts of being beaten, slapped, kicked, or involved in sexual activities
- Precocious sexual behaviors
- Exteme fear or anxiety

Additional signs
- Mistrust of others
- Blunted or flat affect
- Depression or mood changes
- Social withdrawal
- Lack of appropriate peer relationships
- Sudden school difficulties, such as poor grades, truancy, or fighting with peers
- Nonspecific headaches, stomachaches, or eating and sleeping problems
- Clinging behavior directed toward health care providers
- Aggressive speech or behavior toward adults
- Abusive behavior toward younger children and pets
- Runaway behavior

Making a case

Your role in reporting abuse

As a nurse, you play a crucial role in recognizing and reporting incidents of suspected abuse. While caring for patients, you can readily note evidence of apparent abuse. When you do, you must pass the information along to the appropriate authorities. In many states, failure to report actual or suspected abuse constitutes a crime.

  If you've ever hesitated to file an abuse report because you fear repercussions, remember that the Child Abuse Prevention and Treatment Act protects you against liability. If your report is bona fide (that is, if you file it in good faith), the law protects you from a suit filed by an alleged abuser.

The write stuff

- Record only facts; leave out personal opinions and judgments.
- Record the time and date of the entry.
- Provide a comprehensive history, noting:
  - inconsistencies in histories
  - evasive answers
  - delays in seeking treatment
  - medical attention sought at other hospitals
  - person caring for the individual during the incident.
- Document physical assessment findings, using illustrations and photographs as needed (per police department and social service guidelines).

> Documenting "the write stuff" ensures that you have essential data in your chart.

- Describe the patient's response to interventions.
- Record the names and departments of people notified, including supervisors, social services, police department, and welfare agencies.
  - Record visits by the people or agencies notified.
- Document patient teaching and support given.

06/08/06	1700	Circular burns 2 cm in diameter noted on lower ® and Ⓛ scapulae in various stages of healing while auscultating breath sounds. Pt. states these injuries occurred while playing with cigarettes he found at his babysitter's home. When parents were questioned separately as to the cause of injuries on child's back, mother stated the child told her he fell off a swing and received a rope burn. Father stated he had no idea of the child's injuries. Parents stated the child is being watched after school until they get home by the teenager next door, Sally Strong. Parents stated that their son doesn't like being watched by her anymore, but they don't know why. Parents state they're looking into alternative child care. Dr. Gordon notified of injuries and examined pt. at 1645. Social worker, Ben Stiller, and nursing supervisor, Nancy Taylor, RN, notified at 1650.
		———————————— Joan Allen, RN

Activities of daily living

- Standardized checklists for activities of daily living (ADLs) are completed and signed by the nursing staff and, in some cases, the patient performing the activities.
- These forms tell about the patient's abilities, degree of independence, and special needs so the type of assistance each patient requires can be determined.
- Tools useful for assessing and documenting ADLs include:
  - Katz index
  - Lawton scale
  - Barthel index.

The write stuff

- Include the patient's name, the date and time of the evaluation, and your name and credentials.
- On the Katz index, check whether the patient can perform tasks independently, needs some help to perform tasks, or requires significant help to perform tasks in these six areas:
  - bathing
  - dressing
  - toileting
  - moving from wheelchair to bed and returning
  - continence
  - feeding.

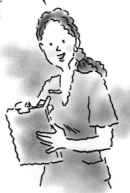

Use the Katz index, Lawton scale, or Barthel index to document ADLs.

- Using the Lawton scale, rate the patient's ability to perform complex personal care activities necessary for independent living using a three-point scale (1 = completely unable to perform task, 2 = needs some help, 3 = performs activity without help) in areas such as:
  - using the telephone
  - cooking or preparing meals
  - shopping
  - doing laundry
  - managing finances
  - taking medications
  - doing housework.
- Using the Barthel index, rate the patient's ability to perform ADLs according to the amount of assistance the patient needs in:
  - feeding
  - moving from wheelchair to bed and returning
  - performing personal hygiene
  - getting on and off the toilet
  - bathing
  - walking on a level surface or propelling a wheelchair
  - going up and down stairs
  - dressing and undressing
  - maintaining bowel continence
  - controlling the bladder.
- The Barthel self-care rating scale evaluates function in more detail.

Form fitting

Barthel index

The Barthel index is used to assess the patient's ability to perform 10 activities of daily living, document findings for other health care team members, and reveal performance improvement or decline.

Date *December 14, 2006*
Patient's name *Joseph Amity*
Evaluator *John Keyburn, RN*

Action	With help	Independent
Feeding (if food needs to be cut = help)	5	⑩
Moving from wheelchair to bed and return (includes sitting up in bed)	5 to ⑩	15
Personal grooming (washing face, combing hair, shaving, cleaning teeth)	0	⑤
Getting on and off toilet (handling clothes, wipe, flush)	⑤	10
Bathing self	0	⑤
Walking on level surface or, if unable to walk, propelling wheelchair	0	⑤ or 15
Ascending and descending stairs	⑤	10
Dressing (includes tying shoes, fastening fasteners)	⑤	10
Controlling bowels	5	⑩
Controlling bladder	⑤	10

DEFINITION AND DISCUSSION OF SCORING
A person scoring 100 is continent, feeds himself, dresses himself, gets up out of bed and chairs, bathes himself, walks at least a block, and can ascend and descend stairs. This doesn't mean that he's able to live alone; he may not be able to cook, keep house, or meet the public, but he's able to get along without attendant care.

Barthel index *(continued)*

Feeding

• 10 = Independent. The person can feed himself a meal from a tray or table when someone puts the food within his reach. He must be able to put on an assistive device, if needed, cut the food, use salt and pepper, spread butter, and so forth. Also, he must accomplish these tasks in a reasonable time.

• 5 = The person needs some help with cutting food and other tasks, as listed above.

Moving from wheelchair to bed and return

• 15 = The person operates independently in all phases of this activity. He can safely approach the bed in his wheelchair, lock brakes, lift footrests, move safely from bed, lie down, come to a sitting position on the side of the bed, change the position of the wheelchair, if necessary, to transfer back into it safely, and return to the wheelchair.

• 10 = Either the person needs some minimal help in some step of this activity, or needs to be reminded or supervised for safety in one or more parts of this activity.

• 5 = The person can come to a sitting position without the help of a second person but needs to be lifted out of bed, or needs a great deal of help with transfers.

Handling personal grooming

• 5 = The person can wash hands and face, comb hair, clean teeth, and shave. He may use any kind of razor but he must be able to get it from the drawer or cabinet and plug it in or put in a blade without help. A woman must put on her own makeup, if she uses any, but need not braid or style her hair.

Getting on and off toilet

• 10 = The person is able to get on and off the toilet, unfasten and refasten clothes, prevent soiling of clothes, and use toilet paper without help. He may use a wall bar or other stable object for support, if needed. If he needs to use a bed pan instead of toilet, he must be able to place it on a chair, use it competently, and empty and clean it.

• 5 = The person needs help to overcome imbalance, handle clothes, or use toilet paper.

Bathing self

• 5 = The person may use a bath tub or shower or give himself a complete sponge bath. Regardless of method, he must be able to complete all the steps involved without another person's presence.

Walking on a level surface

• 15 = The person can walk at least 50 yards without help or supervision. He may wear braces or prostheses and use crutches, canes, or a walkerette, but not a rolling walker. He must be able to lock and unlock braces, if used; get the necessary mechanical aids into position for use; stand up; sit down, and dispose of aids when he sits. (Putting on, fastening, and taking off braces is scored under "Dressing and undressing").

• 5 = If the person can't ambulate but can propel a wheelchair independently, he must be able to go around

(continued)

Barthel index *(continued)*

corners, turn around, maneuver the chair to table, bed, toilet, and other locations. He must be able to push a chair at least 150' (45.7 m). Don't score this item if the person receives a score for walking.
• 0 = Unable to walk.

Ascending and descending stairs
• 10 = The person can go up and down a flight of stairs safely without help or supervision. He may and should use handrails, canes, or crutches when needed, and he must be able to carry canes or crutches as he ascends or descends.
• 5 = The person needs help with or supervision of any one of the above items.

Dressing and undressing
• 10 = The person can put on, fasten, and remove all clothing (including any prescribed corset or braces) and tie shoe laces (unless he requires adaptations for this). Such special clothing as suspenders, loafers, and dresses that open down the front may be used when necessary.
• 5 = The person needs help in putting on, fastening, or removing

any clothing. He must do at least half the work himself and must accomplish the task in a reasonable time. Women need not be scored on use of a brassiere or girdle unless these are prescribed garments.

Controlling bowels
• 10 = The person can control his bowels without accidents. He can use a suppository or take an enema when necessary (as in spinal cord injury patients who have had bowel training).
• 5 = The person needs help in using a suppository or taking an enema or has occasional accidents.

Controlling bladder
• 10 = The person can control his bladder day and night. Spinal cord injury patients who wear an external device and leg bag must put them on independently, clean and empty the bag, and stay dry, day and night.
• 5 = The person has occasional accidents, can't wait for the bed pan or get to the toilet in time, or needs help with an external device.

The total score is less significant or meaningful than the individual items because these indicate where the deficiencies lie. Any applicant to a long-term care facility who scores 100 should be evaluated carefully before admission to see whether admission is indicated. Discharged patients with scores of 100 shouldn't require further physical therapy but may benefit from a home visit to see whether any environmental adjustments are needed.

© Adapted with permission from Mahoney, F.I., and Barthel, D.W. "Functional Evaluation: The Barthel Index," *Maryland State Medical Journal* 14:62, 1965.

Admission assessment form

- Also known as a *nursing database,* the nursing admission assessment form contains the initial patient assessment data.
- Completing the form involves collecting information from various sources and analyzing it to assemble a complete picture of the patient.
- Information obtained can assist with forming nursing diagnoses and creating patient problem lists.
- The nursing admission form may differ among facilities and even among departments in a facility.
- Depending on the form, you may fill in blanks, check off boxes, or write a narrative assessment.
- The form communicates patient information to other health care providers.

The write stuff

- Record:
  - your nursing observations
  - the patient's perception of his health problems
  - the patient's health history
  - your physical examination findings.
- Include these data:
  - current use of prescription and over-the-counter drugs
  - allergies to foods, drugs, and other substances
  - ability to perform activities of daily living
  - support systems
  - cultural and religious information
  - patient's expectations of treatment
  - status of the patient's advance directive.

Form fitting

Completing the nursing admission assessment

Most health care facilities use a combined checklist and narrative admission form such as the one below. The nursing admission assessment becomes a part of the patient's permanent medical record.

ADMISSION DOCUMENT
(To be completed on or before admission by an RN)

Name: _David Connors_
Age: _74_
Birth date: _4/15/31_
Address: _3401 Elm Ave._
Jenkintown, PA
Hospital I.D. No.: _4227_
Insurer: _Aetna_
Policy No.: _605310P_
Physician: _Joseph Milhouse_
Admission date: _1/28/06_

Preoperative teaching
according to standard? ☐ Yes ☑ No
Preoperative teaching completed on
_____

If no, ☑ Surgery not planned
☐ Emergency surgery

Signature _Kate McCauley, RN_

T _101°_   P _120_   R _24_
BP (Lying/sitting) Left: _124/66_
Right: _120/68_

Height: _5'7"_   Weight: _160_

Admitted from:
☐ Emergency department
☐ Home
☑ Doctor's office
☐ Transfer from _____
Mode:
☐ Ambulatory ☑ Wheelchair
☐ Stretcher Accompanied by: _Wife_

Pulses:
L: _P_ Radial _P_ DP _P_ PT
R: _P_ Radial _P_ DP _P_ PT
Apical pulse: _120_
☑ Regular ☐ Irregular
P = Palpable   D = Doppler   O = Absent

Completing the nursing admission assessment *(continued)*

Medical and surgical history
Asthma, type 2 diabetes, high cholesterol

Chief complaint
Shortness of breath

Physical assessment

	Within normal limits	Interviewer comments
Neurological		
Level of consciousness	✓	
Oriented	✓	
Psychosocial		
Behavior	✓	
Coping	✓	
Visual/Auditory	☐	_Wears glasses_
Cardiovascular		
Heart rhythm	✓	
Rate	✓	
Edema	☐	_2 + LE_
Pulses	☐	_1 + LE_
Respiratory		
Rate	✓	
Lungs clear	☐	_Mild wheezes on inspiration_
Dyspnea	☐	_Denies_
Gastrointestinal		
Abdomen soft	✓	
Bowel sounds	✓	
Diet	☐	_Diabetic_
Genitourinary		
Voids	✓	
Urine	✓	

	Within normal limits	Interviewer comments
Musculoskeletal		
Range of motion	✓	
Gait	✓	
Joints	☐	_Knee pain_
Deficits	✓	
Skin		
Temperature	✓	
Turgor	✓	
Pressure ulcers	☐	_None present_
Wounds	☐	_None present_
Pain		
Location	☐	_Knees_
Intensity/Quality (1-10)	☐	_0 – 4_
When started	☐	_3 months ago_
What helps	☐	_Ibuprofen_

List any surgeries the patient has had:

Date	Type of surgery

UNIT INTRODUCTION

Patient rights given to patient: ✓ Y ☐ N
Patient verbalizes understanding: ✓ Y ☐ N
✓ Patient ✓ Family oriented to:
  Nurse call system/unit policies: ✓ Y ☐ N
  Smoking/visiting policy/intercom/siderails/TV channels: ✓ Y ☐ N

Patient valuables:
✓ Sent home
☐ Placed in safe
☐ None on admission

Patient meds:
✓ Sent home
☐ Placed in pharmacy
☐ None on admission

(continued)

Completing the nursing admission assessment *(continued)*

Allergies or reactions
Medications/dyes ☑Y ☐N *PCN — hives*
Anesthesia drugs ☐Y ☑N
Foods ☐Y ☑N
Environmental (eg: tape, latex, bee stings,
 dust, pollen, animals, etc.) ☑Y ☐N *Dust, pollen, cats*

Advance directive information
1. Does patient have health care power of attorney? _____ ☐Y ☑N
 Name _____ Phone _____
 If yes, request copy from patient/family and place in chart
 Date done _____ Init. _____
2. Does patient have a living will? ☑Y ☐N
3. Educational booklet given to patient/family? ☐Y ☑N
4. Advise attending physician if there is a living will
 or power of attorney ☑Y ☐N

Organ and tissue donation
1. Has patient signed an organ and/or tissue donor card? ☑Y ☐N
 If yes, request information and place in chart. Date done *1/28/06*
 If no, would patient like to know more about
 the subject of donation? ☐Y ☐N
2. Has patient discussed his wishes with family? ☑Y ☐N

Medications
Does patient use any over the counter Aspirin ☐Y ☑N
medications? Laxatives ☑Y ☐N
 Vitamins ☑Y ☐N
 Weight loss ☐Y ☑N

What does the patient usually take for minor pain relief? *Acetaminophen*

Prescribed medication (presently in use)	Reason	Dose	Last time taken
1. *Proventil*	Asthma	2 puffs q4hr	1/27/06
2.			
3.			
4.			

Signature *Kate McCauley, RN* Date *1/28/06*

Advance directive

- An advance directive is a legal document that guides life-sustaining medical care and end-of-life decisions when a patient with an advanced disease or disability is no longer able to indicate his own wishes.
- Two types of advance directives are:
  - living will, which instructs practitioners regarding life-sustaining treatment decisions
  - durable power of attorney for health care, a legal document that names a health care proxy (a person to act on the patient's behalf for medical decisions in the event that the patient can't act for himself).
- If a patient has an advance directive, request a copy for the chart and notify the practitioner.
- Be aware that laws for creating advance directives vary by state and advance directives from one state may not be recognized by another state.
- Psychiatric evaluation is usually required for a legal determination of lack of capacity.

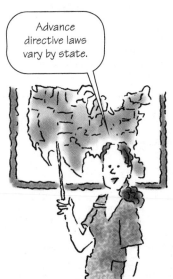

Advance directive laws vary by state.

The write stuff

- Document the presence of an advance directive and the name of the practitioner notified.
- Record the name, address, and telephone number of the person entrusted with decision-making.

Form fitting

Advance directive checklist

The Joint Commission on Accreditation of Healthcare Organizations requires that information on advance directives be charted on the admission assessment form. However, many facilities also use checklists like the one shown here.

ADVANCE DIRECTIVE CHECKLIST   **Patient:** _Eric Landers_

I. Distribution of advance directive information

    A. Advance directive information was presented to the patient: .... ☐
        1. At the time of preadmission testing .... ☐
        2. Upon inpatient admission .... ☐
        3. Interpretive services contacted .... ☐
        4. Information was read to the patient .... ☐
    B. Advance directive information was presented to the next of
    kin as the patient is incapacitated .... ☐
    C. Advance directive information wasn't distributed as the patient
    is incapacitated and no relative or next of kin was available .... ☐

II. Assessment of advance directive upon admission	Upon admission		Upon transfer to Critical Care Unit	
	Yes	No	Yes	No
A. Does the patient have an advance directive?	☑	☐	☐	☐
If yes: Was the attending physician notified?	☑	☐	☐	☐
Was a copy placed in the patient's chart?	☑	☐	☐	☐
B. If he has no advance directive, does the patient want to execute an advance directive?	☐	☐	☐	☐
If yes, was the attending physician notified?	☐	☐	☐	☐
Was the patient referred to resources?	☐	☐	☐	☐

III. Receipt of an advance directive after admission

    A. The patient has presented an advance directive after admission
    and the attending physician has been notified.

Dorothy Terry, RN   _7/07/06_
RN   Date

- Indicate that you read the advance directive and have forwarded it to the appropriate department for review.
- If the patient's wishes differ from those of his family or practitioner, document the discrepancies.
- If a patient doesn't have an advance directive, document that he was given written information concerning his rights under state law to make decisions regarding his health care.
- If the patient refuses information about an advance directive, document this refusal using the patient's own words in quotes.
- Document conversations with the patient regarding his decision making.
- If the patient's capacity is being questioned, document when proof of competence is obtained (usually the responsibility of the medical, legal, social services, or risk management department).

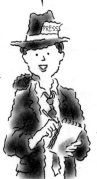

Always quote your source when documenting that a patient refused information about an advance directive.

| 07/07/06 | 1000 | Pt. admitted with advance directives. Dr. Wellington notified at 0950 about living will and durable power of attorney. Copy of advance directives read and placed in medical record, and copy forwarded to Melissa Edwards in Risk Management. Mary Gordon, pt.'s daughter, has durable power of attorney for health care (123 Livingston Drive, Newton, VT, phone: 123-456-7890). ———— Dorothy Terry, RN |

Adverse drug effects

- An adverse drug effect (also called a *side effect*) is an undesirable response that may be mild, severe, or life-threatening.
- Reporting adverse drug effects helps ensure the safety of drugs regulated by the Food and Drug Administration (FDA).
- Complete an FDA MedWatch form when you suspect that a drug is responsible for:
  - death
  - life-threatening illness
  - initial or prolonged hospitalization
  - disability
  - congenital anomaly
  - need for medical or surgical intervention to prevent a permanent impairment or an injury.
- Promptly inform the FDA of product quality problems, such as:
  - defective medication delivery devices
  - inaccurate or unreadable product labels
  - packaging or product mix-ups
  - intrinsic or extrinsic contamination or stability problems
  - particulates in injectable drugs
  - product damage.
- When filing a MedWatch form, you aren't expected to establish a connection between the drug and the problem; you only have to report the adverse event or the problem with the drug.

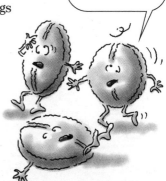

If we're acting adversely, immerse yourself in a MedWatch form.

- Send completed forms to the FDA by using the fax number or mailing address on the form.
- For voluntary reporting, nurses can also report adverse events online using the MedWatch Voluntary Reporting Online Form (3500).
- The mandatory reporting MedWatch form (3500a) may be downloaded but can't be submitted online.
- Remember to comply with your health care facility's protocols for reporting adverse events associated with drugs.
- Product lot numbers are used in product identification, tracking, and product recall.
  - The lot number should be retained.
  - Your supervisor should keep a copy of the report on file.
- The FDA will report back to you on the actions it takes.

The write stuff

- When completing a MedWatch form, include:
  - patient information
  - whether an adverse event, a product problem, or both occurred
  - date of the event
  - description of the event
  - relevant tests or history
  - drug information (including name, dose, frequency, route, and lot number)
  - device information (including type of device, brand, model or serial number, operator of the device, and whether the device is available for evaluation)
  - your name and whether you want your identity as the reporter disclosed.

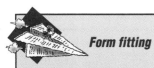

Form fitting

Medwatch form for reporting adverse drug effects

MEDW**ATCH**
THE FDA MEDICAL PRODUCTS REPORTING PROGRAM

For **VOLUNTARY** reporting by health professionals of adverse events and product problems

Page _1_ of _1_

Form Approved: OMB No. 0910-0291 Expires: 4/30/96
See OMB statement on reverse

FDA Use Only
Triage unit sequence #

A. Patient information

1. Patient identifier	2. Age at time of event: or Date of birth:	3. Sex	4. Weight
01234 In confidence	3/11/58	☑ female ☐ male	___ lbs or 59. kgs

B. Adverse event or product problem

1. ☐ Adverse event and/or ☑ Product problem (e.g., defects/malfunctions)

2. Outcomes attributed to adverse event (check all that apply)
- ☐ death _____ (mo/day/yr)
- ☐ life-threatening
- ☐ hospitalization – initial or prolonged
- ☐ disability
- ☐ congenital anomaly
- ☐ required intervention to prevent permanent impairment/damage
- ☐ other:

3. Date of event 3/8/06

4. Date of this report 3/8/06

5. Describe event or problem

After reconstituting 100-mg vial with 10 ml of bacteriostatic water, the drug crystallized and turned yellow.

Drug wasn't given.

PLEASE TYPE OR USE BLACK INK

6. Relevant tests/laboratory data, including dates

7. Other relevant history, including preexisting medical conditions (e.g., allergies, race, pregnancy, smoking and alcohol use, hepatic/renal dysfunction, etc.)

C. Suspect medication(s)

1. Name (give labeled strength & mfr/labeler, if known)
#1 *Leucovorin calcium for injection—*
#2 *100-mg vial*

2. Dose, frequency & route used	3. Therapy dates (if unknown, give duration) from/to (or best estimate)
#1 100 mg IV X1	#1 3/8/06
#2	#2

4. Diagnosis for use (indication)
#1 *Megaloblastic anemia*
#2

5. Event abated after use stopped or dose reduced
#1 ☐ yes ☐ no ☐ doesn't apply
#2 ☐ yes ☐ no ☐ doesn't apply

6. Lot # (if known)	7. Exp. date (if known)
#1 #891	#1
#2	#2

6. Event reappeared after reintroduction
#1 ☐ yes ☐ no ☐ doesn't apply
#2 ☐ yes ☐ no ☐ doesn't apply

9. NDC # (for product problems only)
–

10. Concomitant medical products and therapy dates (exclude treatment of event)

D. Suspect medical device

1. Brand name

2. Type of device

3. Manufacturer name & address

4. Operator of device
- ☐ health professional
- ☐ lay user/patient
- ☐ other:

5. Expiration date (mo/day/yr)

6. model #

catalog #

serial #

lot #

other #

7. If implanted, give date (mo/day/yr)

8. If explanted, give date (mo/day/yr)

9. Device available for evaluation? (Do not send to FDA)
☑ yes ☐ no ☐ returned to manufacturer on _____ (mo/day/yr)

10. Concomitant medical products and therapy dates (exclude treatment of event)

E. Reporter (see confidentiality section on back)

1. Name & address phone # (123) 456-7890
Patricia Cohen
987 Cedargrove Lane
Cincinnati, Ohio

2. Health professional? ☑ yes ☐ no

3. Occupation RN

4. Also reported to
- ☐ manufacturer
- ☐ user facility
- ☑ distributor

5. If you do NOT want your identity disclosed to the manufacturer, place an "X" in this box. ☐

FDA Mail to: MEDWATCH or FAX to:
5600 Fishers Lane 1-800-FDA-0178
Rockville, MD 20852-9787

FDA Form 3500 1/96 Submission of a report does not constitute an admission that medical personnel or the product caused or contributed to the event.

Against medical advice discharge

- A patient may decide to leave a health care facility against medical advice (AMA). Possible reasons a patient may leave AMA include:
  - he doesn't understand his condition or treatment
  - he has pressing personal problems
  - he wants to exert control over his health care
  - he has religious or cultural objections to his care
  - he's dissatisfied with his medical care or the facility.
- The law requires clear evidence that a patient is mentally competent to choose to leave the health care facility AMA.
- In most facilities, an AMA form (also known as a *responsibility release form*) protects you, the practitioners, and the facility if problems arise from a patient's unapproved discharge.
- Make sure the patient is contacted in a timely manner with pending test results.
- Provide routine discharge care because your patient's rights to discharge planning and care are the same as a patient who has signed out with medical advice.
- If the patient allows it, escort him to the door (in a wheelchair, if necessary), arrange for medical or nursing follow-up care, and offer other routine health care measures.

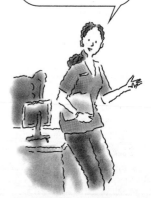

You should provide discharge planning even if the patient signs out against medical advice.

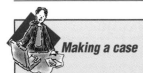

Making a case

Patient discharge against medical advice

The patient's bill of rights and the laws and regulations based on it give a competent adult the right to refuse treatment for any reason without being punished or having his liberty restricted. Some states have turned these rights into law, and the courts have cited the bill of rights in their decisions. The right to refuse treatment includes the right to leave the hospital against medical advice (AMA) any time, for any reason. As a nurse, your only recourse is to try to talk the patient out of leaving.

If your patient still insists on leaving AMA and your hospital has a policy on managing the patient who wants to leave, follow it exactly. Adhering to policy helps to protect the hospital, your coworkers, and you from charges of unlawful restraint or false imprisonment.

The write stuff

- Have the patient or legal guardian sign the AMA form.
- Include in your notes:
  - patient's reason for leaving AMA
  - that the patient knows he's leaving AMA
  - names of relatives or others notified of the patient's decision and the dates and times of the notifications
  - date and time the practitioner was notified
  - time of practitioner's visit with the patient
  - instructions or orders given by the practitioner
  - explanation of the risks and consequences of the AMA discharge, as told to the patient, including the name of the person who provided the explanation
  - instructions regarding alternative sources of follow-up care given to the patient
  - names of those accompanying the patient at discharge and the instructions given to them

Form fitting

Responsibility release form

An against medical advice form, or responsibility release form, is a medical record as well as a legal document. It's designed to protect you, your coworkers, and your institution from liability resulting from the patient's unapproved discharge.

Responsibility release

This is to certify that I, _Robert Brown_ ,

a patient in _Jefferson Memorial Hospital_ ,

am being discharged against the advice of my doctor and the hospital admin- istration. I acknowledge that I have been informed of the risk involved and hereby release my doctor and the hospital from all responsibility for any ill effects that may result from such a discharge. I also understand that I may return to the hospital at any time and have treatment resumed.

Robert Brown   _11/4/06_
[Patient's signature]   [Date]

Carl Giordano, MD   _11/4/06_
[Witness' signature]   [Date]

RE: _Robert Brown_   Patient identification # _123456_
[Name of patient]

    – patient's destination and contact information after dis- charge so that he can be informed of pending test results.
- Document statements and actions reflecting the patient's mental state at the time he chose to leave the facility.
- Fill out an incident report, if your facility requires it, for a patient who leaves without anyone's knowledge or if a pa- tient refuses to sign the AMA form.
- If a patient refuses to sign the AMA form, document this re- fusal on the AMA form using the patient's own words.

11/04/06	1500	Pt. found in room packing his clothes. When
		asked why he was dressed and packing, he
		stated, "I'm tired of all these tests. They keep
		doing tests, but they still don't know what's
		wrong with me. I can't take anymore. I'm going
		home." Dr. Giordano notified and came to speak
		with pt. Doctor told pt. of possible risks and
		consequences of his leaving the hospital with
		headaches and hypertension. Pt. agreed to
		see Dr. Giordano in his office in 2 days.
		Prescriptions given to pt. Pt.'s wife was
		notified and came to the hospital. She was
		unable to persuade husband to stay. Pt. signed
		AMA form. Discussed low-sodium diet, meds,
		and appt. with pt. and wife. Gave pt. drug
		information sheets. Pt. will call for pending
		test results. Pt. states he's going home after
		discharge. Accompanied pt. in wheelchair to
		main lobby with wife. Pt. left at 1445. ——————
		————————————————— Vickie Vale, RN

Anaphylaxis

- A severe reaction to an allergen after reexposure to the substance, anaphylaxis is potentially fatal and requires emergency intervention.
- If airway, breathing, and circulation become compromised, cardiopulmonary resuscitation may be necessary.
- Monitor vital signs frequently.
- If the cause is immediately evident, perform appropriate interventions; for example, for a transfusion reaction:
  - stop the infusion
  - change the tubing
  - keep the I.V. line open with a normal saline solution infusion.
- Contact the practitioner immediately and anticipate orders, such as administering an epinephrine injection.
- When the patient is stable, perform an assessment to identify the cause of the anaphylactic reaction.

The write stuff

- Document the date and time that the anaphylactic reaction started.
- Record the events leading up to the anaphylactic response.
- Document the patient's signs and symptoms, such as anxiety, agitation, flushing, palpitations, itching, chest tightness, light-headedness, throat tightness or swelling, throbbing in the ears, or abdominal cramping.
- Document how soon after allergen exposure signs and symptoms started.
- Include assessment findings, such as arrhythmias, rash, wheals or welts, wheezing, decreased level of consciousness, unresponsiveness, angioedema, hypotension, weak or rapid pulse, edema, and diaphoresis.

- Note the name of the practitioner notified, time of notification, emergency treatments and supportive care given, and the patient's response.
- If the allergen is identified, follow facility protocol and note it on the medical record, medication administration record, nursing care plan, patient identification bracelet, practitioner's orders, and dietary and pharmacy profiles.
- Document the departments and individuals notified, including the pharmacy, the dietary department, risk management, and the nursing supervisor.
- Fill out an incident report form, if indicated.

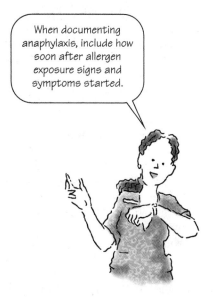

09/01/06	1545	Pt. received Demerol 50 mg I.M. for abdominal
		incision pain at 1510. At 1520 pt. became SOB
		and diaphoretic and c/o intense itching
		"everywhere." Injection site on Ⓛ buttock has
		4-cm erythematous area. Skin is blotchy and
		upper anterior torso and face are covered
		with hives. BP 90/50, P 140 and regular, RR 44
		in semi-Fowler's position. I.V. of D₅ ½NSS
		infusing at 125 ml/hr in Ⓛ hand. Exp. wheezes
		heard bilaterally. O₂ sat. 94% via pulse oximetry
		on room air. O₂ at 4 L/min via NC started with
		no change in O₂ sat. Pt. alert and oriented
		to time, place, and person but anxious and
		restless. Dr. Brown notified of pt.'s symptoms
		at 1525 and orders implemented. Fluid
		challenge of 500 ml NSS over 60 min via Ⓛ
		antecubital began at 1535. O₂ changed to 50%
		humidified face mask with O₂ sat. increasing to
		99%. After 15 min of fluid challenge, BP 110/70,
		P 104, RR 28. Benadryl 25 mg P.O. given for
		discomfort after fluid challenge absorbed.
		Allergy band placed on pt.'s Ⓛ hand for possible
		Demerol allergy. Chart, MAR, nursing care plan,
		and doctor's orders labeled with allergy
		information. Pharmacy, dietary dept., and
		nursing supervisor, Betty Rubble, RN, notified.
		Pt. told he had what appeared to be an allergic
		reaction to Demerol, that he shouldn't receive
		it in the future, and that he should notify all
		health care providers and pharmacies of this
		reaction. Recommended that pt. wear a medical
		ID bracelet noting his allergic reaction to
		Demerol. Medical ID bracelet order form given
		to pt.'s wife. ——————— Arvin Sloan, RN

Note: the ½NSS and subscript notations appear as D_5 ½NSS in the original. The O₂ references appear as O_2.

Arrhythmias

- An abnormal electrical conduction or automaticity of the heart's intrinsic pacemaker produces changes in the heart rate, rhythm, or both.
- Arrhythmias vary in severity from mild, asymptomatic disturbances requiring no treatment to catastrophic ventricular fibrillation, which requires immediate resuscitation.
- Arrhythmias are classified according to their origin (atrial, ventricular, or junctional).
- Clinical significance depends on the effect on cardiac output and blood pressure.
- Prompt detection and intervention can mean the difference between life and death.

The write stuff

- Record the date and time of the arrhythmia.
- Document events before and at the time of the arrhythmia.
- Record the patient's symptoms and cardiovascular assessment findings, such as pallor, cold and clammy skin, shortness of breath, palpitations, weakness, chest pain, dizziness, syncope, and decreased urine output.
- Include vital signs and heart rhythm.
- If the patient is on a cardiac monitor, place a rhythm strip in the chart.
- Note the name of the practitioner notified, time of notification, and any orders received.
- If ordered, report the results of a 12-lead electrocardiogram.

> If the patient is on a cardiac monitor, place a rhythm strip in the chart.

- Document interventions performed and the patient's response.
- Record the emotional support and patient teaching given.

| 05/24/06 | 1700 | While assisting pt. with ambulation in the hallway at 1640, pt. c/o feeling weak and dizzy. Pt. said he was "feeling my heart hammering in my chest." Pt. stated he never felt like this before. Apical rate 170; BP 90/50; RR 24; peripheral pulses weak; skin cool, clammy, and diaphoretic. Denies chest pain or SOB. Breath sounds clear bilaterally. Pt. placed in wheelchair and assisted back to bed without incident. O_2 via NC started at 2 L/min. Dr. Brown notified at 1645 and orders noted. Lab called to draw stat serum electrolyte and digoxin levels. Stat ECG revealed PSVT at a rate of 180. I.V. infusion of D_5W started in Ⓛ hand at 30 ml/hr with 18G cannula. Placed pt. on continuous cardiac monitoring with portable monitor from crash cart. At 1650 apical rate 180, BP 92/52, pulses weakened in all 4 extremities, lungs clear, skin cool and clammy. Pt. still c/o weakness and dizziness. Pt. transferred to telemetry unit. Report given to Lotte Schwartz, RN. Nursing supervisor, Carol Malkovich, RN, notified. —— Cathy Keener, RN |

Arterial line insertion

- An arterial line permits continuous measurement of systolic, diastolic, and mean pressures as well as arterial blood sampling.
- Direct arterial monitoring is indicated when highly accurate or frequent blood pressure measurements are required.
- Obtain informed consent if required by your facility.
- An Allen's test must be performed before insertion.
- Using sterile technique, a preassembled kit is used to prepare and anesthetize the insertion site.
- The catheter is inserted in the artery by the practitioner and attached to fluid-filled tubing and a pressure bag.

The write stuff

- Record the results of the Allen's test.
- Record the name of the practitioner inserting the arterial line.
- Include the time and date of insertion.
- Note the insertion site, the size and length of the catheter, and whether the catheter is sutured in place.

Did somebody say Allen's test?

- Document systolic, diastolic, and mean pressure readings upon insertion, and include a monitor strip of the waveform.
- Record circulation in the extremity distal to the insertion site by assessing color, pulses, and sensation.
- Include the amount of flush solution infused every shift.
- Document the emotional support and patient teaching given.

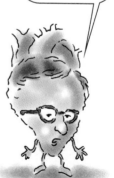

09/05/06	0625	#20G 2½" arterial catheter placed in ® radial
		artery by Dr. Mayer on second attempt after a
		+ Allen's test. Catheter secured with 1 suture.
		Transparent dressing applied. ® hand and
		wrist secured to arm board. Transducer leveled
		and zeroed. Good waveform on monitor. Initial
		readings 92/64, mean arterial pressure
		73.3 mm Hg with pt. in semi-Fowler's position.
		Readings accurate to cuff pressures. Site
		without redness or swelling. ® hand pink, warm,
		with 2-sec. capillary refill. No c/o numbness or
		tingling. Line flushes easily. Pt. told to call
		nurse for numbness, tingling, pain, or coolness
		in ® hand. Pt. verbalized understanding. ————
		————————————— Milo Zed, RN

Jones, Raymond   ICU 04A   9/5/06   0625

Arterial line removal

- An arterial line is removed when it's no longer necessary or the insertion site needs to be changed.
- Consult your facility's policy to determine whether registered nurses are permitted to perform this procedure and follow procedure as outlined by your facility's policy.

The write stuff

- Record the time and date the catheter is removed.
- Include the name of the person removing the catheter.
- Document the length of the catheter, condition of the insertion site, and the reason why the catheter is being removed.
- Note if catheter specimens were obtained for culture.
- Record how long pressure was maintained to control bleeding.
- Include the type of dressing applied.
- Document circulation in the extremity distal to the insertion site, including color, pulses, and sensation, and compare findings to the opposite extremity.
- Document neurovascular checks as your facility's policy states.

03/07/06	1200	Arterial catheter removed from Ⓡ radial site
		by the RN. Pressure applied for 10 min.
		Insertion site without bruising, swelling, or
		hematoma. Sterile gauze dressing with povidone-
		iodine ointment applied. BP 102/74, P 84,
		RR 16, oral T 99.7° F. Catheter tip sent to
		laboratory for culture and sensitivity. Ⓡ and Ⓛ
		hands warm and pink. Radial pulse strong. Pt
		has no c/o numbness, tingling, or pain in Ⓡ or
		Ⓛ hand. Will continue to check circulation to Ⓡ
		hand according to orders.— *Lisa Chang, RN*

Arterial pressure monitoring

- Arterial pressure monitoring permits continuous measurement of systolic, diastolic, and mean pressures.
- This type of monitoring is indicated when:
  - highly accurate or frequent blood pressure measurements are required, such as for patients with low cardiac output and high systemic vascular resistance or patients who receive titrated vasoactive drugs
  - patients require frequent blood sampling.
- A frequent vital signs assessment sheet may be used to record repeated measurements.

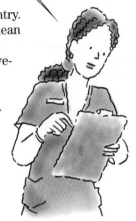

When it comes to insertion sites, appearances count. Include a description of the site in your chart.

The write stuff

- Record the date and time of each entry.
- Document systolic, diastolic, and mean arterial pressure readings.
- Describe the appearance of the waveform, and include a monitor strip.
- Include a comparison with an auscultated blood pressure reading.
- Record circulation in the extremity distal to the site, including color, warmth, capillary refill, pulses, pain, movement, and sensation.
- Describe the appearance of the insertion site, noting evidence of infection or bleeding.
- Note whether tubing or flush solution is changed.
- Document dressing changes and site care performed.
- Document recalibration of the equipment.

- Include the amount of flush solution infused in your note as well as on the intake and output record.

| 09/06/06 | 0500 | BP 90/60, MAP 70, via ® radial arterial line, with pt. at 45-degree angle. Cuff BP 86/58. Monitor shows normal arterial waveform. See strip mounted below. ® hand warm, pink, with capillary refill less than 3 sec. Pt. able to move fingers of ® hand, no c/o pain, able to feel light touch. No redness, tenderness, warmth, drainage, or bleeding noted at insertion site. Dressing removed. Tubing and flush solution changed. Dry, sterile dressing applied. ® wrist immobilizer reapplied, no skin breakdown noted. 30 ml of flush solution used this shift. ————————— Abigail Lockhart, RN |

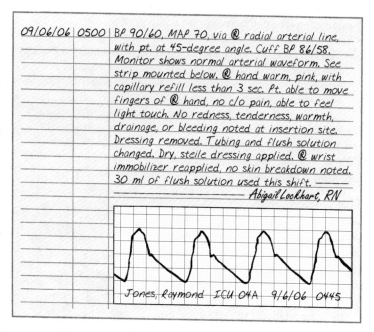

Jones, Raymond   ICU 04A   9/6/06   0445

B

Blood transfusion

- Blood transfusion involves the replacement of whole blood or a blood component, such as packed cells, plasma, platelets, or cryoprecipitates, to compensate for losses caused by surgery, trauma, or disease.
- Proper identification and crossmatching procedures must be performed before the transfusion to ensure the correct patient receives the correct blood product.
- The transfusion may be administered when:
  - identification and crossmatching information are confirmed
  - consent form has been signed
  - patient's vital signs have been obtained and abnormal findings, such as elevated temperature, have been reported.

The write stuff

- Before administering a blood transfusion, document that two licensed health care professionals, according to facility policy, matched the label on the blood bag at the patient's bedside to the:
  - patient's name
  - patient's identification number
  - patient's blood group or type

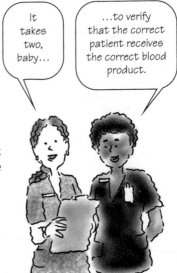

It takes two, baby...

...to verify that the correct patient receives the correct blood product.

- patient's and donor's Rh factor
- crossmatch data
- blood bank identification number
- expiration date of the product.
- On the transfusion record, document:
  - date and time that the transfusion was started and completed
  - names and credentials of the health care professionals who verified the information
  - type and gauge of the infusion catheter and insertion site
  - total amount of the transfusion
  - patient's vital signs before, during, and after the transfusion, according to facility policy
  - infusion device used (if any) and its flow rate
  - blood-warming unit used (if any)
  - amount of normal saline solution used (if any)
  - patient's response to the transfusion.
- If the patient receives his own blood, document the amount of blood retrieved and reinfused in the intake and output records.
- Document laboratory data during and after the autotransfusion, including:
  - coagulation profile
  - hematocrit and hemoglobin level
  - arterial blood gas study results
  - calcium levels.

02/13/06	1015	Pt. to be transfused with 1 unit of PRBCs over
		4 hr, according to written orders of Dr. Mays.
		Label on the blood bag checked by me and
		Nancy Gallager, RN, who verified the following
		information on the blood slip: 1 unit PRBCs for
		George Andrews, #123456, pt. and donor O+,
		Rh+ compatible crossmatch, blood bank #54321,
		expiration date 12/23/06. Consent form signed
		by pt. ———————————— Monica Belinski, RN
02/13/06	1030	Infusion of 1 unit of PRBCs started at 1025
		through 18G catheter in Ⓛ forearm at 15 ml/hr
		using blood transfusion tubing. P 82, BP 132/84,
		RR 16, oral T 98.2° F. Remained with pt. for
		first 15 min. and increased rate to 60 ml/hr.
		———————————— Monica Belinski, RN
02/13/06	1045	No c/o itching, chills, wheezing, or headache. No
		evidence of vomiting, swelling, laryngeal edema,
		or fever noted. PRBCs increased to 63 ml/hr.
		P 84, BP 128/82, RR 17, oral T 97.9° F. ———
		———————————— Monica Belinski, RN
02/13/06	1430	Transfusion of 1 unit PRBCs complete. P 78, BP
		130/78, RR 16, oral T 98.0° F. No c/o itching,
		chills, wheezing, or headache. No evidence of
		vomiting, swelling, laryngeal edema, or fever
		noted. ———————————— Monica Belinski, RN

Blood transfusion reaction

- During a blood transfusion, the patient is at risk for developing a transfusion reaction.
- If a reaction develops, immediately:
  - stop the transfusion
  - take down the blood tubing
  - hang new tubing with normal saline solution running to maintain vein patency
  - notify the practitioner, blood bank, and laboratory
  - complete a transfusion reaction form
  - follow facility policy for a blood transfusion reaction.

The write stuff

- Document the time and date of the reaction.
- Record the name of the practitioner you notified, the time of notification, any orders received, supportive care given, and the patient's response.
- Record the time you notified the blood bank, the name of the person with whom you spoke, and directions received.
- Include the type and amount of infused blood or blood products.
- Note the time the transfusion was started and the time it was stopped.
- Record clinical signs of the reaction in order of occurrence.
- Include the patient's vital signs.
- Document urine specimens or blood samples sent to the laboratory for analysis.

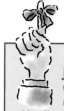

Memory jogger

When documenting a blood transfusion reaction, include the "five times":

Time and date of the reaction

Time the doctor was notified

Time the blood bank was notified

Time the transfusion was started

Time the transfusion was stopped.

Form fitting

Transfusion reaction report

If your facility requires a transfusion reaction report, you'll include the following types of information.

TRANSFUSION REACTION REPORT   **Name:** *Graham Stoker*

Nursing report

1. Stop transfusion immediately. Keep I.V. line open with saline infusion.
2. Notify responsible practitioner.
3. Check all identifying names and numbers on the patient's wristband, unit, and paperwork for discrepancies.
4. Record patient's posttransfusion vital signs.
5. Draw posttransfusion blood samples (clotted and anticoagulated), avoiding mechanical hemolysis.
6. Collect posttransfusion urine specimen from patient.
7. Record information as indicated below.
8. Send discontinued bag of blood, administration set, attached I.V. solutions, and all related forms and labels to the blood bank with this form completed.

Clerical errors

☑ None detected
☐ Detected

Vital signs

	Pre-TXN	Post-TXN
Temp.	98.4°	97.6°F
B.P.	120/60	160/88
Pulse	88	104

Assessment findings

☐ Urticaria   ☐ Perspiration
☑ Fever   ☐ Shock
☐ Chills   ☐ Oozing
☐ Chest pain   ☐ Back pain
☐ Hypotension   ☐ Infusion site pain
☐ Nausea   ☐ Hemoglobinuria
☐ Flushing   ☐ Oliguria or anuria
☐ Dyspnea   ☐ Cyanosis of lips noted
☐ Headache

Reaction occurred

During administration? *Yes*
After administration? _____
How long? _____
Medications added? *No*
Previous I.V. fluids? *NSS at 30 ml/hr*
Blood warmed? *No*

Specimen collection

Blood: Difficulty collecting? *No*
Urine: Voided *Yes, sent to lab*
       Catheterized _____

Comments:
Given diphenhydramine 50 mg I.M.

Signature *Monica Belinski, RN*   **Date** *2/13/06*

- Indicate that you sent the blood transfusion equipment (discontinued bag of blood, administration set, attached I.V. solutions, and all related forms and labels) to the blood bank.
- Complete a transfusion reaction report, according to facility policy, and send it to the blood bank.
- Document your follow-up care.

02/13/06	1400	Pt. reports chills. Cyanosis of lips noted at
		1350. Transfusion of packed RBCs stopped.
		Approximately 100 ml of blood infused.
		Transfusion started at 1215, stopped at 1350.
		Tubing changed. I.V. of 1000 ml NSS infusing
		at 30 ml/hr rate in ® forearm. Notified Dr.
		Cahill at 1353 and John Adams in blood bank at
		1355. BP 168/88, P 104, RR 25, rectal T 97.6° F.
		Two red-top tubes of blood drawn from pt.
		and sent to lab. Urine specimen obtained from
		catheter. Urine specimen sent to lab for U/A.
		Administered diphenhydramine 50 mg I.M. per
		Dr. Cahill's order. Two blankets placed on pt.
		Blood transfusion equipment sent to blood
		bank. Transfusion reaction report filed. ——
		—————————————— Monica Belinsky, RN
02/13/06	1415	Pt. reports he's getting warmer. BP 148/80,
		P 96, RR 20, T 97.6° F. —— Monica Belinsky, RN
02/13/06	1430	Pt. no longer complaining of chills. I.V. of
		1000 ml NS infusing at 125 ml/hr in ® arm.
		BP 138/76, P 80, RR 18, T 98.4° F. ——
		—————————————Monica Belinsky, RN

Brain death

- Brain death is commonly defined as the irreversible cessation of all brain function, including the brain stem.
- Know your state's laws regarding the definition of brain death as well as your facility's policy. The Uniform Determination of Death Act guides the principles of making a diagnosis of brain death.
- American Academy of Neurology (AAN) guidelines recommend that at least one doctor examine the patient to confirm the presence of the three cardinal signs of brain death:
  - coma, including suspected cause and whether it's reversible
  - absence of brain stem function
  - apnea.
- The patient is tested for responsiveness or movement, brain stem reflexes (pupillary, corneal, gag and cough, oculocephalic, and oculovestibular), and apnea.
- Laboratory and diagnostic test results are used to eliminate other causes of coma.
- The AAN recommends examination on two separate occasions at least 6 hours apart by two doctors; the second doctor shouldn't be involved in the patient's care.

The write stuff

- Document family teaching and emotional support provided.
- Record the date and time of the examination and the name of the person performing the test.
- Include your observation of the patient's response.
- Record the time of brain and cardiopulmonary death, and include evidence such as electrocardiogram strips.

> Don't be afraid to name names. Including the names of others involved in the patient's care makes for a complete chart.

06/01/06	0800	Dr. Malone in to speak with pt.'s son, Mark Newton, who has health care POA, about pt.'s condition. Son verbalized understanding about probable brain death due to subarachnoid hemorrhage. Son agreed to tests to determine brain death. Son was teary and spent a few minutes verbalizing about his father's good qualities. When offered, stated he didn't want a visit by clergy or social worker. ———————————————————— *Susan Orlean, RN*
06/01/06	0815	Dr. Malone performed clinical exam. See Physical Progress Notes for full report. Son present for exam. Dr. Malone explained to son pt.'s lack of response and absence of reflexes. Son understands that another Dr. not involved with his father's care will repeat the exam in 6 hours. ———————————— *Susan Orlean, RN*
06/01/06	0830	ABG results obtained by Joanne Burke, RPT, with pt. on ventilator. Results pH 7.40, PO_2 100, PCO_2 40. Pt. taken off ventilator by respiratory therapist and placed on 100% O_2 via T-piece. Dr. Malone in attendance. Cardiac monitor showing NSR at a rate of 70, O_2 sat. via continuous pulse oximetry 99%. Within 1 minute of testing, heart rate 150 with PVCs, and O_2 sat. dropped to 91%. Pt. without spontaneous respirations. ABGs drawn by respiratory therapist showed pH 7.32, PO_2 60, PCO_2 65. Pt. placed back on ventilator. Son verbalized understanding of the results showing apnea. Son states he will stay with his dad until exam at 1430 with Dr. Porter. Dr. Malone will meet with son at 1500 to discuss results and plan. ———————— *Susan Orlean, RN*

C

Cardiac monitoring

- Cardiac monitoring allows continuous observation of the heart's electrical activity.
- It's used to:
  - assess cardiac rhythm
  - gauge a patient's response to drug therapy
  - prevent complications associated with diagnostic and therapeutic procedures.
- Electrodes that transmit electrical signals are placed on the patient's chest.
- The electrical signals are converted into a tracing of cardiac rhythm on an oscilloscope.
- Types of cardiac monitoring include:
  - hardwire monitoring, in which the patient is connected to a monitor at bedside
  - telemetry, in which a small transmitter connected to the patient sends an electrical signal to a monitor screen for display.

The write stuff

- Document the date and time that monitoring began.
- Indicate the monitoring leads used.
- Place a rhythm strip in the chart and label it with the patient's name, the date, and the time.

> Don't be misleading. Record the leads used during cardiac monitoring in the chart.

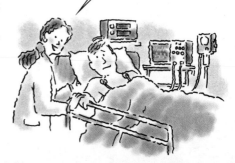

- Record the PR interval, QRS duration, and QT interval, along with an interpretation of the rhythm.
- Document changes in the patient's condition.
- If cardiac monitoring will continue after the patient's discharge, document which caregivers can interpret dangerous rhythms and can perform cardiopulmonary resuscitation.
- Document all patient and caregiver teaching, such as troubleshooting techniques to use if the monitor malfunctions.
- Note referrals (for example, to equipment suppliers).

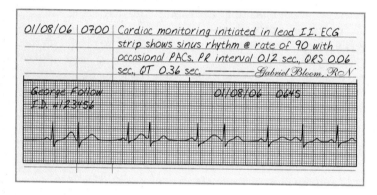

| 01/08/06 | 0700 | Cardiac monitoring initiated in lead II. ECG strip shows sinus rhythm @ rate of 90 with occasional PACs. PR interval 0.12 sec., QRS 0.06 sec., QT 0.36 sec. ——— Gabriel Bloom, RN |

George Follow
I.D. #123456   01/08/06   0645

Cardiac tamponade

- In cardiac tamponade, a rapid, unchecked rise in intrapericardial pressure impairs diastolic filling of the heart.
- This condition is usually caused by increased pressure from blood or fluid accumulation in the pericardial sac.
- Rapid fluid accumulation requires emergency lifesaving measures.
- Cardiac tamponade may:
  - be idiopathic (Dressler's syndrome)
  - result from effusion, hemorrhage from trauma or nontraumatic causes, pericarditis, acute myocardial infarction, chronic renal failure during dialysis, drug reaction, or connective tissue disorders.
- If cardiac tamponade is suspected, notify the practitioner immediately and prepare for pericardiocentesis (needle aspiration of the pericardial cavity), emergency surgery (usually a pericardial window), or both.
- Anticipate I.V. fluids, inotropic drugs, and blood products to maintain blood pressure until treatment is performed.

The write stuff

- Note the date and time that signs of tamponade began.
- Include assessment findings, such as jugular vein distention, decreased arterial blood pressure, pulsus paradoxus, narrow pulse pressure, muffled heart sounds, acute pain, dyspnea, diaphoresis, anxiety, restlessness, pallor or cyanosis, rapid and weak pulses, and hepatomegaly.
- Record the name of the practitioner notified, the time of notification, and any orders received.
- Note the diagnostic tests ordered by the practitioner, such as an electrocardiogram, an echocardiogram, or a chest X-ray, and their findings.

- Document the treatments and procedures performed and the patient's response to them.
- Note patient teaching and emotional support given.
- Document vital signs, drug titration, and patient responses on the appropriate flow sheets.

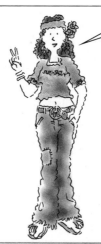

Go with the flow sheets, man.

| 06/05/06 | 1320 | BP at 1300 90/40 via cuff on ® arm. Last BP at 1245 was 120/60. Drop of 17 mm Hg in systolic BP noted during inspiration. P 132 and regular, RR 34, oral T 97.2° F. See frequent vital sign sheet for q15min VS. Neck veins distended with pt. in semi-Fowler's at 45-degrees, heart sounds muffled, peripheral pulses weak. Pt. anxious and dyspneic. Skin pale and diaphoretic. Pt. c/o chest soreness from MVA and hitting steering wheel. Slight ecchymosis visible across chest. Pt. awake, alert, and oriented to time, place, and person. Dr. Olsen notified at 1305. Stat portable CXR shows slightly widened mediastinum and enlargement of the cardiac silhouette. ECG shows sinus tachycardia with rate of 130. 200-ml bolus of NSS given. Dopamine 400 mg in 250 D₅W started via distal port of ® subclavian TLC at 4 mcg/kg. Urine output is 25 ml for last hr. Awaiting Dr. Olsen's arrival for pericardiocentesis. Explained the procedure to pt. and wife and answered their questions. Consent obtained. ————— _Cindy Brady, RN_ |

Cardiopulmonary arrest and resuscitation

- American Heart Association guidelines call for a written, chronological account of a patient's condition throughout cardiopulmonary resuscitation (CPR).
- The code record is a precise, quick, and chronological recording of the events of the code.
- The designated recorder's role during the code is to document therapeutic interventions and the patient's responses.
- A resuscitation critique form is commonly used to:
  - identify actual or potential problems with the resuscitation process
  - track personnel responses and response times
  - track the availability of appropriate drugs and functioning equipment.

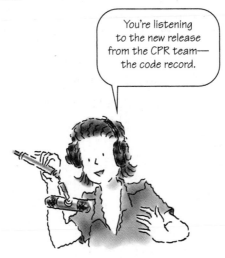

You're listening to the new release from the CPR team— the code record.

Form fitting

The code record

The code record *(continued)*

Pg. _2_ of _2_

ABGs and LAB DATA							
Time spec sent	pH	PCO	Po₂	HCO₃⁻	Sat%	Fio₂	Other
0635	7.1	76	43	14	80%		

Resuscitation outcome

☑ Successful
☑ Transferred to _CCU_ at _0648_
☐ Unsuccessful – Expired at_____
Pronounced by: _____MD
Family notified by: _S. Quinn, RN_
Time: _0645_
Attending notified by: _S. Quinn, RN_
Time: _0645_
Code recorder _S. Quinn, RN_
Code Team Nurse _B. Mullen, RN_
Anesthesia Rep. _J. Hanna, RN_
Other personnel _Dr. Barbera_
_____B. Russo, RT

The write stuff

- Document the date and time the code was called.
- Record the patient's name, location of the code, the person who discovered the patient, the patient's condition, and whether the arrest was witnessed or unwitnessed.
- Record the name of the practitioner notified, time of notification, and names of other members who participated in the code.
- On the code record, note the exact time for each code intervention and include:
  - vital signs
  - heart rhythm
  - laboratory results (such as arterial blood gas or electrolyte levels)
  - treatment given (such as CPR, defibrillation, or cardioversion)
  - drugs given (name, dosage, and route)
  - procedures performed (such as intubation, transvenous pacemaker insertion, and central line insertion)
  - patient response.

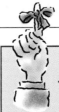

- Record the time that the family was notified.
- Indicate the patient's status at the end of the code and the time the code ended.
- If required by the facility, the practitioner leading the code and the nurse recording the code must review the code sheet and sign it.
- Record in the nurse's notes:
  - events leading up to the code
  - assessment findings prompting you to call a code
  - who initiated CPR
  - interventions performed before the code team arrived
  - patient's response to interventions
  - that a code sheet was used to document the events of the code.

Memory jogger

When documenting a code, use the mnemonic **WE CARE** to help remember what to include in your notes:

Who initiated cardiopulmonary resuscitation

Events leading up to the code

Care provided before code team arrived

Assessment findings prompting the code

Response of patient to interventions

Events documented in a code sheet.

| 11/09/06 | 0650 | Summoned to pt.'s room at 0630 by a shout from roommate. Found pt. unresponsive in bed without respirations or pulse. Roommate stated, "He was talking to me; then all of a sudden he started gasping and holding his chest." Code called at 0630. Initiated CPR with Ann Barrow, RN. Code team arrived at 0632 and continued resuscitative efforts. (See code record.) ———————————————— Connie Brown, RN |

Cardioversion, synchronized

- Synchronized cardioversion involves delivery of an electric charge to the myocardium at the peak of the R wave, causing immediate depolarization, interrupting reentry circuits, and allowing the sinoatrial node to resume control.
- Synchronizing the low-energy shock with the R wave ensures that the current won't be delivered on the vulnerable T wave, disrupting repolarization.
- Indications include unstable tachyarrhythmias associated with organized QRS complexes and pulses, unstable supraventricular tachycardia, atrial fibrillation, atrial flutter, and unstable monomorphic ventricular tachycardia with a pulse.
- Cardioversion may be an elective or urgent procedure, depending on how well the patient tolerates the arrhythmia.

The write stuff

- Document the date and time of the cardioversion.
- Record whether a consent form was signed.
  - If the need for the procedure is urgent, document that the situation didn't allow for obtaining consent.
- Document patient teaching given and the patient's response.
  - If the need for the procedure is urgent, document that the situation didn't allow for patient teaching.
- Include preprocedure activities, such as withholding food and fluids, withholding drugs, removing dentures, administering a sedative, and obtaining a 12-lead electrocardiogram (ECG).
- Document vital signs. Obtain a rhythm strip before starting.
- Note that the synchronized setting was used, the voltage used, and the number of times the patient was cardioverted.
- After the procedure, record vital signs, place a rhythm strip in the chart, and note that a 12-lead ECG was obtained and the results.
- Document the patient's recovery, including level of consciousness, airway patency, respiratory rate and depth, and use of supplemental oxygen until he's awake.

- Indicate the specific time of each assessment; avoid block charting.

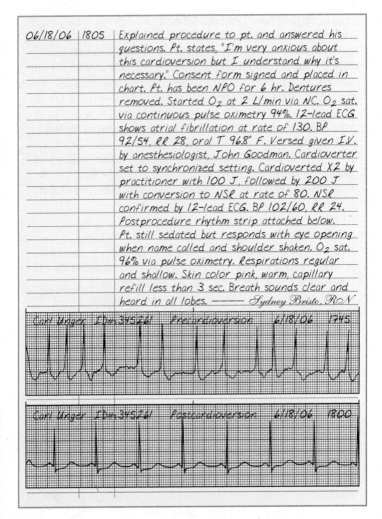

06/18/06 | 1805 | Explained procedure to pt. and answered his questions. Pt. states, "I'm very anxious about this cardioversion but I understand why it's necessary." Consent form signed and placed in chart. Pt. has been NPO for 6 hr. Dentures removed. Started O_2 at 2 L/min via NC. O_2 sat. via continuous pulse oximetry 94%. 12-lead ECG shows atrial fibrillation at rate of 130. BP 92/54, RR 28, oral T 96.8° F. Versed given I.V. by anesthesiologist, John Goodman. Cardioverter set to synchronized setting. Cardioverted X2 by practitioner with 100 J, followed by 200 J with conversion to NSR at rate of 80. NSR confirmed by 12-lead ECG. BP 102/60, RR 24. Postprocedure rhythm strip attached below. Pt. still sedated but responds with eye opening when name called and shoulder shaken. O_2 sat. 96% via pulse oximetry. Respirations regular and shallow. Skin color pink, warm, capillary refill less than 3 sec. Breath sounds clear and heard in all lobes. ——— Sydney Bristo, RN

Carl Unger ID#345261 Precardioversion 6/18/06 1745

Carl Unger ID#345261 Postcardioversion 6/18/06 1800

Central venous catheter insertion

- A sterile catheter is inserted through a major vein, such as the subclavian vein or jugular vein.
- A central venous catheter is used:
  - for central venous pressure monitoring (which indicates blood volume or pump efficiency)
  - for aspiration of blood samples
  - for administration of I.V. fluids (in large amounts, if necessary) in emergencies
  - when decreased peripheral circulation causes peripheral veins to collapse
  - when prolonged I.V. therapy reduces the number of accessible peripheral veins
  - when solutions must be diluted (for large volumes or for irritating or hypertonic fluids such as total parenteral nutrition solutions)
  - when long-term venous access is needed.
- A peripherally inserted central catheter (PICC) is inserted in a peripheral vein, such as the basilic vein, and is used for infusion and blood sampling only.

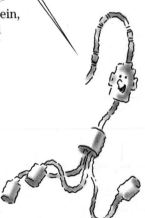

Don't you forget about me. Document my type, length, and location.

The write stuff

- Document the time and date of central line insertion.
- Record the name of the practitioner inserting the line.
- Note the type, length, and location of the catheter.
- Include the solution being infused.

- Record the patient's response to the procedure.
- If the ports aren't being used for continuous infusion, document that the ports have needle-free injection caps and include orders related to maintaining patency.
- Document the time the X-ray was performed to confirm placement, the location of the catheter tip, and your notification of the practitioner.
- Note whether the catheter is sutured in place and the type of dressing applied.
- For a PICC, record the length of the external catheter.

02/24/06	2300	Procedure explained to pt. and consent obtained by Dr. Chavez. Pt. in Trendelenburg's position and 20.3 cm central line catheter placed by Dr. Chavez on first attempt in Ⓡ subclavian vein. Cath sutured in place with 3-0 silk, and sterile dressing applied per protocol. Needle-free injection caps placed on all lines. Lines flushed with 100 units heparin. Portable CXR obtained to confirm line placement. Results pending. P 110, BP 90/58, RR 24, oral T 97.9° F. Pt. sitting in semi-Fowler's position and breathing easily, lungs clear bilaterally. —————— Emma Thompson, RN
02/24/06	2350	Received telephone report from Dr. Turner in radiology confirming proper placement of central line tip in superior vena cava. Dr. Chavez notified by phone of report. ———————— Emma Thompson, RN

Central venous catheter removal

- When a central venous (CV) line is no longer necessary, it's removed by the practitioner or by a specially trained nurse.
- Verify your facility's policy and protocols related to CV line removal by a registered nurse.

The write stuff

- Record the name of the person discontinuing the line.
- Include the time and date of the removal.
- Document the length of time that pressure was held to the site.
- Note the length of the catheter and the condition of the insertion site.
- Describe site care and the type of dressing applied.
- Document whether catheter specimens were collected for culture or other analysis.

02/24/06	1100	20.3 cm CV catheter removed by Dr. Romero at
		1045 and pressure held for 5 min. Catheter tip
		present, sent to laboratory for culture.
		Povidone-iodine applied to insertion site and
		covered with gauze pad and transparent
		semipermeable dressing. No drainage, redness,
		or swelling noted at insertion site. ———
		——————————— Diane Court, RN

Central venous catheter site care

- Central venous catheter site care and frequency varies according to the type of catheter, the type of dressing, and facility policy.
- Site care is performed using sterile technique.
- The insertion site should be visually inspected and gently palpated daily through an intact occlusive dressing.
- Assess the site for signs and symptoms of infection, such as discharge, inflammation, and tenderness.
- Dressings should be changed if they become soiled or lose integrity.
- Depending on facility policy, documentation of site care may be in the nurse's notes or on the I.V. therapy flow sheet.

The write stuff

- Record the date and time of site care.
- Note the marking indicating catheter length.
- Describe the appearance of the insertion site.
- Record how the site was cleaned and the type of dressing applied.
- Describe any drainage found on the dressing.
- If complications are noted, record the name of the practitioner notified, the time of notification, and orders received.
- Include patient teaching provided.

10/29/06	1220	® subclavian gauze dressing removed. Suture intact, insertion site without redness or drainage, catheter marking at 12 cm. Pt. denies tenderness. Using sterile technique, area and insertion site cleaned with chlorhexidine. Catheter secured with tape and covered with semipermeable membrane dressing. ———————————— Niles Crane, RN

Change in patient condition

- You must report to the practitioner and document changes in a patient's condition in a timely manner.
- Proper documentation of your conversation with the practitioner is essential to meet patient safety goals and to verify response to a change in condition if a patient's care comes into question.
  - Writing "Notified practitioner of patient's condition" is too vague.

Help desk

Communicating condition changes over the phone

- If you don't know the practitioner, ask him to state and spell his full name.
- Include the exact time you contacted the practitioner. If you don't note the time you called, allegations may be made later that you failed to obtain timely medical treatment for the patient.
- Always note in the chart the specific change, problem, or result you reported to the practitioner, along with the practitioner's orders or response. Use his own words.
- If you're reporting a critical laboratory test result (for example, a serum potassium level of 3.2 mEq/L) but don't receive an order for intervention (such as potassium replacement therapy), be sure to verify with the practitioner that he doesn't want to give an order and document this fact in the progress notes. For example, write: "Dr. Jones informed of potassium level of 3.2 mEq/L. No orders received."
- If you think a practitioner's failure to order an intervention puts your patient's health at risk, follow the chain of command and notify your supervisor. Then be sure to document your action.

- In the event of a malpractice suit, the plaintiff's lawyer (and the practitioner) could imply that you didn't communicate essential data.
- Chart exactly what you told the practitioner.

The write stuff

- Your note should include:
  - date and time that you notified the practitioner
  - practitioner's name
  - what you reported
  - practitioner's response
  - any orders received (if no orders were received, document that also)
  - interventions performed.

| 10/03/06 | 0900 | Pt. had moderate-sized, soft, dark brown stools positive for blood by guaiac test. Abdomen soft and nontender; positive bowel sounds heard in all four quadrants. Skin warm, pink, capillary refill less than 3 sec. P 92, BP 128/68, RR 28, oral T 97.2° F. Dr. Rodriguez notified of findings at 0915. Hemoglobin level and hematocrit added to morning blood work, as ordered. Doctor in to discuss with pt. the need for colonoscopy. Pt. agreed to procedure, which is scheduled for 0800 on 10/04/06. Explained bowel prep procedure to pt. Consent obtained. ———————————— Josie Paterno, RN |

Chest pain

- When your patient complains of chest pain, act quickly to determine its cause.
- Chest pain may be caused by a disorder as benign as epigastric distress (indigestion) or as serious and life-threatening as acute coronary syndrome.

The write stuff

- Record the date and time of the onset of chest pain.
- Document the patient's responses (in his own words, if appropriate) to your questions about his pain, including:
  - what the patient was doing when the pain started
  - how long the pain lasted, if it had ever occurred before, and whether the onset was sudden or gradual
  - whether the pain radiates
  - factors that improve or aggravate the pain
  - exact location of the pain (ask him to point to the pain and record his response)
  - severity of the pain (ask the patient to rank the pain on a 0-to-10 scale, with 0 indicating no pain and 10 indicating the worst pain imaginable).
- Record the patient's vital signs.
- Include your assessment of his body systems.
- Record the name of the practitioner notified, the time of notification, and any orders received.
- Document the time and name of other individuals notified, such as the nursing supervisor or admission's department (if the patient is transferred).
- Record your actions and the patient's responses.
- Include patient teaching and emotional support you provided.

08/09/06	0410	Pt. c/o sudden onset of a sharp chest pain while sleeping. Points to center of chest, over sternum. States, "It feels like an elephant is sitting on my chest." Pain radiates to the neck and shoulders. Rates pain as 7 on a scale of 0 to 10, w/10 being the worst pain imaginable. P 112, BP 90/62, RR 26. Lungs have fine crackles in the bases on auscultation. Dr. Howser notified of findings at 0405 and orders received. Morphine 2 mg I.V. given. O_2 at 4 L/min started by NC. Continuous pulse oximetry started with O_2 sat. 94%. 12-lead ECG and MI profile obtained. All procedures explained to pt. Reassured pt. that he's being closely monitored. ———————— _Martha Wolcott, RN_
08/09/06	0415	Dr. Howser here to see patient. Pt. states pain is now a 5 on a scale of 0 to 10. Morphine 2 mg I.V. repeated. ECG interpreted by Dr. Romano to show acute ischemia. Pt. prepared for transport to CCU. Nancy Holmes, RN, nursing supervisor, notified of transfer. ——— ———————— _Martha Wolcott, RN_

Chest physiotherapy

- Chest physiotherapy includes postural drainage, chest percussion and vibration, and coughing and deep-breathing exercises.
- It's used to move and eliminate secretions, reexpand lung tissue, and promote efficient use of respiratory muscles.
- It also helps prevent or treat atelectasis in bedridden patients and may help prevent pneumonia.

The write stuff

- Document the date and time of chest physiotherapy.
- Record the patient's position for secretion drainage and the length of time the patient remained in each position.
- Note the chest segments percussed or vibrated.
- Describe the characteristics of secretions expelled, including color, amount, odor, viscosity, and presence of blood.
- Record indications of complications, actions taken, and the patient's tolerance of the treatment.
- Include patient teaching provided.

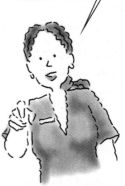

Make it your mission to document the patient's position when draining secretions.

12/20/06	1415	Pt. placed on Ⓛ side with foot of bed elevated.
		Chest PT and postural drainage performed for
		10 min. from lower to middle then upper lobes,
		as ordered. Pt. had productive cough and
		expelled large amt. of thick, yellow, odorless
		sputum. Lungs clear after chest PT. After chest
		PT, pt. stated he was tired and asked to lie
		down. ———————————— Geena Davids, RN

Chest tube care

- Inserted into the pleural space, a chest tube allows blood, fluid, pus, or air to drain and allows the lung to reinflate.
- Chest drainage uses gravity or suction to restore negative pressure and remove material that collects in the pleural cavity.
- An underwater seal in the drainage system allows air and fluid to escape from the pleural cavity but doesn't allow air to reenter.
- Caring for the patient with a chest tube involves:
  – maintaining suction
  – monitoring for and preventing air leaks
  – monitoring drainage
  – promoting pulmonary hygiene
  – promoting patient comfort
  – performing dressing changes and site care, if ordered
  – preventing, detecting, and treating complications.

The write stuff

- Record the date and time of chest tube care.
- Identify the chest tube location.
- Include the type and amount of suction.
- Describe the type, amount, and consistency of drainage.
- Note the presence or absence of bubbling or fluctuation in the water-seal chamber.
- If site care was performed, record the appearance of the site, the type of dressing applied, and any crepitus palpated.
- Document the patient's respiratory status and pulmonary hygiene performed.
- Note the patient's level of pain, comfort measures performed, and the results.
- Include interventions performed to prevent complications.

- If complications occurred, record:
  - name of the practitioner notified
  - time of notification
  - interventions performed
  - results of interventions.

05/31/06	1350	Received pt. from recovery room at 1325. ®
		midaxillary CT with 20 cm of H_2O in Pleur-
		evac suction control chamber. Collection chamber
		has 100 ml of serosanguineous fluid. No clots
		noted. Level of drainage dated and timed.
		Water level fluctuating with respirations in
		water-seal chamber. All CT connections taped,
		and 2 rubber-tipped clamps placed at bedside.
		Dried blood on CT dsg. No crepitus noted.
		Breath sounds clear with diminished sounds in
		® lower lobe. P 98, BP 132/82, RR 28 shallow
		and labored, oral T 99.1° F. Skin pale, warm,
		and dry, mucous membranes pink. O_2 sat. 97%
		on 50% face mask. Pt. c/o aching pain at CT
		site and refused to take deep breaths and
		cough due to pain. Morphine sulfate 2 mg I.V.
		given at 1335. Pt. able to C&DB within 15 min
		after administration. —————————
		————————————— Mary Ann Pfister, R.N

Chest tube insertion

- A chest tube is inserted, under sterile technique, to permit drainage of air or fluid from the pleural space.
- For pneumothorax, the second intercostal space is the usual insertion site because air rises to the top of the intrapleural space.
- For hemothorax or pleural effusion, the sixth, seventh, and eighth intercostal spaces are common insertion sites because fluid settles to the lower levels of the intrapleural space.
- For removal of air and fluid, a chest tube is inserted into a high site as well as a low site.
- After insertion, the chest tube is connected to a thoracic drainage system that removes air, fluid, or both from the pleural space and prevents backflow into that space, promoting lung reexpansion.
- Inserting a chest tube requires close observation of the patient and verification of proper placement.

The write stuff

- Document the date and time of chest tube insertion.
- Note that informed consent was obtained.
- Include the name of the doctor performing the procedure.
- Identify the insertion site and the type of drainage system and suction used.
- Record the presence of drainage and bubbling.
  - Include drainage on the intake and output record.
  - Record the type, amount, and consistency of drainage.
- Document vital signs, auscultation findings, and other respiratory assessments.
- Document whether a chest X-ray was obtained and, if so, the results.
- Document complications and nursing actions taken.
- Record patient teaching provided.
- Record the patient's tolerance of the procedure.

09/30/06	1100	Pt. consented to insertion of chest tube after
		discussing risks and complications with Dr. Brown.
		Informed consent signed. Preinsertion P 98,
		RR 32, BP 118/72, oral T 97.9° F. Assisted Dr.
		Brown with sterile insertion of #22 CT into
		pt.'s Ⓛ lower midaxillary area. Tube secured
		with one suture. CT connected to Pleur-evac
		with 20 cm of suction, which immediately
		drained 100 ml of serosanguineous drainage.
		No air leaks evident with the system. Post-
		insertion P 80, RR 24, BP 120/72. Respirations
		shallow, unlabored. Slightly decreased breath
		sounds in Ⓛ post. lower lobe, otherwise breath
		sounds clear bilaterally. O_2 sat. 99% after CT
		insertion. Equal lung excursion noted. No
		crepitus palpated. Petroleum jelly gauze applied
		to CT insertion site and occlusive dressing
		applied. Tubing secured to pt. to prevent
		dislodgment. Pt. reports only minimal discomfort
		at insertion site. Upright portable CXR obtained
		immediately after procedure. Dr. Brown
		notified to view results. C&DB exercises and
		use of incentive spirometer reviewed with pt.;
		pt. verbalized understanding and was able to
		inspire 900 ml of volume. — *Ingrid Manberg, RN*

Chest tube removal

- After the patient's lung has reexpanded, the practitioner removes the chest tube.
- In many facilities, other health care professionals such as advanced practice nurses (clinical nurse specialists or nurse practitioners) are trained to perform chest tube removal.

The write stuff

- Document the date and time of chest tube removal and the name of the person who performed the procedure.
- Record the patient's vital signs and the findings of your respiratory assessment before and after chest tube removal.
- Note whether an analgesic was administered before the removal and how long after administration the chest tube was removed.
- Describe the patient's tolerance of the procedure.
- Record the amount of drainage in the collection bottle and the appearance of the wound at the chest tube site.
- Describe the type of dressing applied.
- Document patient teaching performed.

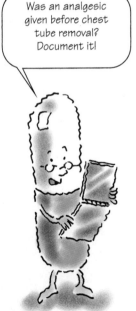

Was an analgesic given before chest tube removal? Document it!

10/09/06	1300	Explained to pt. that CT was being removed
		because Ⓛ lung is now reexpanded. Explained
		how to perform Valsalva's maneuver when tube
		is removed. Pt. was able to give return
		demonstration. Administered Percocet 2 tabs
		P.O. 30 min before removal. Preprocedure
		P 88, BP 120/80, RR 18, oral T 97.8° F.
		Respirations regular, deep, unlabored. No use
		of accessory muscles. Full respiratory excursion
		bilaterally. Breath sounds clear bilaterally. No
		drainage in collection chamber since 0800. #20
		CT removed without difficulty by Dr. Smith.
		CT wound clean. No drainage or redness
		noted. Petroleum jelly gauze dressing placed
		over insertion site, covered with 4" X 4" gauze
		dressing, and secured with 2" tape. Post-
		procedure breath sounds remain clear, full
		respiratory excursion bilaterally, breathing
		comfortably in semi-Fowler's position, no
		subcutaneous crepitus noted. P 86, BP 132/84,
		RR 20. Pt. without c/o pain or SOB. Reminded
		him of importance of continuing to use
		incentive spirometer q1hr. CXR performed at
		1255. Results not yet available. ————————
		—————————————— _Lisa Stock, RN_

Cold application

- Cold application:
  - constricts blood vessels
  - inhibits local circulation, suppuration (pus formation), and tissue metabolism
  - relieves vascular congestion
  - slows bacterial activity in infections
  - reduces body temperature
  - may act as a temporary anesthetic during brief, painful procedures.
- Because treatment with cold also relieves inflammation, helps to prevent edema, and slows bleeding, it may provide effective initial treatment after eye injuries, strains, sprains, bruises, muscle spasms, and burns.

The write stuff

- Record the time, date, and duration of cold application.
- Document the site of application, noting that the device wasn't placed directly on the patient's skin.
- Include the type of device used, such as an ice bag or collar, K pad, cold compress, or chemical cold pack.
- Indicate the temperature or temperature setting of the device.

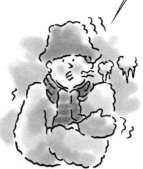

I know that c-c-cold application c-c-can be beneficial. I just c-c-can't remember how right now.

- Before and after the procedure, record the patient's vital signs and the appearance of his skin.
- Document signs of complications, interventions, and the patient's response.
- Describe the patient's tolerance of treatment.
- Include patient teaching provided.

11/14/06	1300	Before cold application, oral T 98.6° F, BP
		110/70, P 80, RR 18. ® groin site warm and dry,
		without redness, edema, or ecchymosis. Reason
		for cold application explained to pt. Ice bag
		covered with towel applied to ® groin for 20
		min. Postprocedure T 98.6° F, BP 120/70, P 82,
		RR 20. ® groin site cool and dry, without
		redness, edema, graying, mottling, blisters, or
		ecchymosis. No c/o burning or numbness. Pt. is
		resting comfortably. ———— Greg Granberg, RN

Communicable disease reporting

- The Centers for Disease Control and Prevention, the Occupational Safety and Health Administration, the Joint Commission on Accreditation of Healthcare Organizations, and the American Hospital Association all require health care facilities to document and report certain diseases acquired in the community or in hospitals and other health care facilities.
- Be aware that reporting laws vary by state.
- Generally, the facility's infection control department reports diseases to the appropriate local authorities who notify the state health department, which in turn reports the diseases to the appropriate federal agency or national organization.

Reportable communicable diseases

According to the Centers for Disease Control and Prevention (2005), certain diseases must be reported to local health authorities. Because regulations vary among communities and states and because different agencies focus on different data, the list of reportable diseases that appears below isn't conclusive and may change periodically.

- Acquired immunodeficiency syndrome (AIDS)
- Anthrax
- Arboviral neuroinvasive and nonneuroinvasive diseases
  - California serogroup virus disease
  - Eastern equine encephalitis virus disease
  - Powassan virus disease
  - St. Louis encephalitis virus disease
  - West Nile virus disease
  - Western equine encephalitis virus disease
- Botulism (foodborne, infant, other)
- Brucellosis
- Chancroid
- Cholera
- Coccidioidomycosis
- Cryptosporidiosis
- Cyclosporiasis
- Diphtheria

Reportable communicable diseases *(continued)*

- Ehrlichiosis (human granulocytic, human monocytic, human, other or unspecifed)
- Giardiasis
- Gonorrhea
- Haemophilus influenzae, invasive disease
- Hansen disease (leprosy)
- Hantavirus pulmonary syndrome
- Hemolytic uremic syndrome, postdiarrheal
- Hepatitis, viral, acute (A, B, B perinatal, C)
- Hepatitis, viral, chronic (B, C past or present)
- Human immunodeficiency virus (HIV) infection
- Influenza-associated pediatric mortality
- Legionellosis
- Listeriosis
- Lyme disease
- Malaria
- Measles
- Meningococcal disease
- Mumps
- Pertussis
- Plague
- Poliomyelitis, paralytic
- Psittacosis
- Q Fever
- Rabies
- Rocky Mountain spotted fever
- Rubella or rubella congenital syndrome
- Salmonellosis
- Severe acute respiratory syndrome-associated coronavirus (SARS-CoV) disease
- Shiga-toxin-producing *Escherichia coli*
- Shigellosis
- Smallpox
- Streptococcal disease, invasive, group A
- Streptococcal toxic shock syndrome
- *Streptococcus pneumoniae*, drug resistant, invasive disease
- Syphilis (primary, secondary, latent, neurosyphilis, congenital)
- Tetanus
- Toxic shock syndrome
- Trichinellosis (trichinosis)
- Tuberculosis
- Tularemia
- Typhoid fever
- Vancomycin—intermediate *Staphylococcus aureus* (VISA)
- Vancomycin—resistant *Staphylococcus aureus* (VRSA)
- Varicella (morbidity)
- Varicella (deaths only)
- Yellow fever

The write stuff

- Document the date, time, and person or department notified (according to your facility's policy and procedure manual).
- Record what you reported.

08/01/06	1400	Notified Ms. Smith, Infectious Disease
		Coordinator of West Brook Memorial Hospital,
		that the diagnosis of West Nile encephalitis
		has been identified as per Dr. John Jones,
		Infectious Disease. ——— Tammy Hartwell, RN

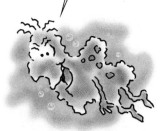

Don't forget to communicate to the proper authorities when your patient has a reportable communicable disease.

Correction to documentation

- When you make a mistake on a chart, correct it promptly.
- Never erase, cover, completely scratch out, or otherwise obscure an erroneous entry because this may imply a cover-up.
  - If the chart ends up in court, the plaintiff's attorney will be looking for anything that may cast doubt on the chart's accuracy.
  - Erasures or the use of correction fluid or heavy black ink to obliterate an error are red flags.

The write stuff

- When you make a mistake documenting on the medical record, correct it by drawing a single line through it and writing the words "mistaken entry" or "error" above or beside it.
  - Make sure the mistaken entry is still readable.
  - Doing so indicates that you're only trying to correct a mistake, not cover it up.
- Follow the "mistaken entry" note with your initials and the date and time.
- If appropriate, briefly explain the need for the correction.

		Mistaken entry. J.M. 1/19/06 0905
01/19/06	0900	~~Pt. walked to bathroom. States he experienced~~
		~~no difficulty urinating.~~ *John Mora, RN*

Critical value reporting

- According to the Joint Commission on Accreditation of Healthcare Organizations' (JCAHO's) 2005 National Patient Safety Goals, critical test results must be reported to a responsible licensed caregiver in a timely manner so that immediate action may be taken.
- Critical test results (as defined by the facility) may include diagnostic tests, such as imaging studies, electrocardiograms, laboratory tests, and other diagnostic studies.
- Because these results influence immediate treatment decisions, report critical test results verbally (either in person or by telephone) to the responsible practitioner.
- Critical test values may be reported to another individual (such as a nurse, unit secretary, or doctor's office staff) who will then immediately report the values to the practitioner or responsible licensed caregiver.
- In instances where a facility doesn't define a set of critical tests, JCAHO considers all verbal and telephone reports of diagnostic tests to be critical.

The write stuff

- Document:
  - the date and time you received the critical test result
  - person who gave the results to you
  - name of the test and the critical value
  - the name of the practitioner or responsible health care provider you notified
  - time of the notification
  - means of communication used
  - orders received.
- If the message wasn't given directly to the licensed practitioner, include confirmation that the critical test result was to be relayed to the practitioner immediately.
- Note instructions or information given to the patient.

- If the message was given to a nurse, unit secretary, or office staff personnel, include that individual's name.

06/04/06	1000	Nanette Lange called from laboratory at 0945 to report critical PT value of 52 seconds. Results reported by telephone to Dr. Potter at 0948, orders given to hold warfarin, obtain PT level in a.m., and call Dr. Potter with results. Pt. informed about elevated PT and the need to hold warfarin until PT levels drop to therapeutic range. Pt. instructed to report any bleeding to nurse. ———— *Penny Lane, RN*

Cultural needs

- Your patient's cultural behaviors and beliefs may be different than your own.
  - Most people in the United States make eye contact when talking with others.
  - People in a number of cultures—including Native Americans, Asians, and people from Arab-speaking countries—may find eye contact disrespectful or aggressive.
- Identifying your patient's cultural needs is the first step in developing a culturally sensitive care plan.
- Depending on your facility's policy, cultural assessment may be part of the admission history form or there may be a separate, more in-depth cultural assessment tool.

The write stuff

- Record the date and time of your assessment.
- Note the patient's communication style:
  - Can he speak and read English?
  - Does he have the ability to read lips?
  - What's his native language?
  - Is an interpreter required?
- Document his nonverbal communication style for eye contact, expressiveness, and ability to understand common signs.
- Record social orientation, including culture, race, ethnicity, family role function, work, and religion.

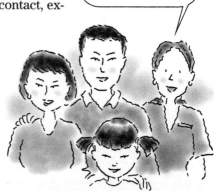

Documenting a patient's cultural needs helps develop a culturally sensitive care plan.

- Document the patient's spatial comfort level, particularly in light of his conversation, proximity to others, body movement, and space perception.

Form fitting

Identifying your patient's cultural needs

A transcultural assessment tool can help promote cultural sensitivity in any nursing setting. Consult your facility's policy on the use of such forms, or incorporate the information included in this sample form when developing your client's care plan.

Date: _3/12/06_ Time: _1015_
Pt. name _Claudette Valiente_ Age _34_ ☐ M ☑ F
Medical dx: _36 weeks pregnant, states "high sugar in my blood"_

COMMUNICATION (language, voice quality, pronunciation, use of silence and nonverbals)

Subjective data
Can you speak English? ☑ Yes ☐ No _____
Can you read English? ☑ Yes ☐ No _With difficulty_
Are you able to read lips? ☐ Yes ☑ No _____
Native language? _Creole_
Do you speak or read any other language? _No_
How do you want to be addressed? ☐ Mr. ☐ Mrs. ☐ Ms.
   ☑ First name ☐ Nickname _____

Objective data
How would you characterize the nonverbal communication style? _Very open_
Eye contact: ☐ Direct
   ☑ Peripheral gaze or no eye contact preferred during interactions
Use of interpreter: ☐ Family ☐ Friend ☐ Professional
   ☐ Other ☑ None
Overall communication style: ☑ Verbally loud and expressive
   ☐ Quiet, reserved ☐ Use of silence
Meaning of common signs — O.K., got ya nose, index finger summons, V sign, thumbs up: _Understands above signs except "got ya nose"_
Determine any familial colloquialisms used by individuals or families that may impact on assessment, treatment, or other interventions. _None noted_

(continued)

Identifying your patient's cultural needs *(continued)*

SOCIAL ORIENTATION (culture, race, ethnicity, family role function, work, leisure, church, and friends)

Subjective data
Country of birth? __Haiti__ Years in this country? _3_
(If an immigrant or a refugee, how long has the patient lived in this country? — You are not questioning citizen status.)
What setting did you grow up in? ☐ Urban ☐ Suburban ☑ Rural
What is your ethnic identity? __Haitian__
What is your race? __Black__
Who are the major support people: ☑ Family members
☐ Friends ☐ Other_____
Who are the dominant family members? __Husband, grandparents__
Who makes major decisions for the family? __A family meeting is held__
Occupation in native country: __None__ Present occupation: __None__
Education? __Finished 6th grade__
Is religion important to you? __Yes__
What is your religious affiliation? __Catholic__
Would you like a chaplain visit? ☐ Yes ☑ No
Any cultural/religious practices/restrictions? If yes, describe __Balancing "hot"__
__and "cold," believes in some voodoo passed down from mother__
__and grandmother__

Objective data
Interaction with family/significant other — describe __Animated, physically__
__close, frequent touch, eye contact with family members__
Age and life cycle factors must be considered in interactions with individuals and families (for example, high value placed on the decision of elders, the role of the eldest man or woman in families, or roles and expectation of children within the family). __Elders highly respected, children expected__
__to be obedient and respectful__
Religious icons on person or in room? __Wearing cross__

SPACE (comfort in conversation, proximity to others, body movement, perception of space)
__Use of touch, kissing, and close proximity with family__

Subjective data
__Distance maintained from nurse and doctor__
Do you have any plans for the future? __No, believes God will guide her__
What do you consider a proper greeting? __Kissing and touch with family__

Objective data
☑ Tactile relationships, affectionate and embracing ☐ Non-contact
Personal space? __Very close with family, maintains 2-3 foot__
__distance from RN__

Identifying your patient's cultural needs *(continued)*

BIOLOGICAL VARIATIONS (skin color, body structure, genetic and enzymatic patterns, nutritional preferences and deficiencies)

Subjective data
What type of food do you prefer? *Rice, beans, plantains*
What type of food do you dislike? *Yogurt, cottage cheese*
What do you believe promotes health? *Good spiritual habits, balancing "hot" and "cold," and eating well*
Family history of disease? *Malaria, high blood pressure, "sugar"*

Objective data
Skin color: *Deep brown*   Hair type: *Coarse*

ENVIRONMENTAL CONTROL (health practices, values, definitions of health and illness)

Subjective data
What do you think caused your problem? *"Ate wrong foods."*
Do you have an explanation for why it started when it did? *"No."*
What does your sickness do to you; how does it work? *"I don't think anything is wrong, but the doctor does."*
How severe is your sickness? How long do you think it will last? *"It will go away soon."*
What problems has your sickness caused you? *"The doctor says my baby is big, but a big baby is a strong baby."*
What fears do you have about your sickness? *"I have no fear. I will have a healthy baby."*
What kind of treatment do you think you should receive? *"Eating healthy."*

What are the most important results you hope to receive from this treatment? *"A healthy baby."*
What are the health and illness beliefs and practices of the family? *Uses home remedies such as herbs to treat sickness*
What are the most important things you do to keep healthy? *"Eat well."*

Any concerns about health and illness? *"No."*

What types of healing practices do you engage in (hot tea and lemon for cold, copper bracelet for arthritis, magnets)? *"Avoiding spices because they bother the baby, balancing hot and cold."*

(continued)

Identifying your patient's cultural needs *(continued)*

ENVIRONMENTAL CONTROL *(continued)*

Objective data
Describe patient's appearance and surroundings: _Patient is clean and neatly groomed. Appears slightly overweight._
What diseases/disorders are endemic to the culture or country of origin? _Intestinal problems, malnutrition, STDs, TB, sickle cell anemia, htn, cancer, AIDS_
What are the customs and beliefs concerning major life events? _"Pregnant women are treated special. Father of the baby doesn't participate in the birth experience; this is 'women's business'."_

TIME (use of measures, definitions, social and work time, time orientation — past, presentt, and future)

Subjective data
Preventative health measures? ☐ Yes ☑ No

Objective data
Time orientation ☐ Present ☑ Past
History of noncompliance, missed appointments? _Often misses appts or arrives late_

Julie McCoy, RN

Source: Victor M. Fernandez, RN, BSN, and Kathy Fernandez, RN, BSN. © 2006 (TC18082)

- Note his skin color and body structure.
- Ask about food preferences, family health history, religious and cultural health practices, and definitions of health and illness.
- Determine the patient's time orientation (past, present, or future).

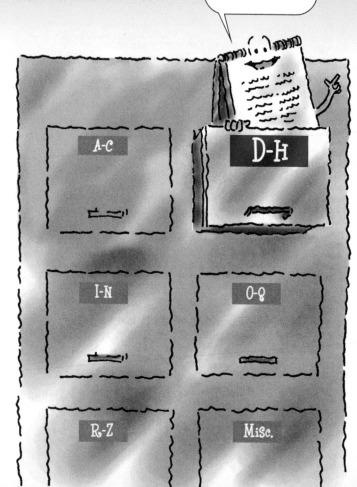

D

Death

- Postmortem care usually begins after a practitioner certifies the patient's death.
- Care includes:
  - preparing the patient for family viewing
  - arranging transportation to the morgue or funeral home
  - determining the distribution of the patient's belongings
  - comforting and supporting the patient's family and friends and providing them with privacy.
- If the patient died violently or under suspicious circumstances, postmortem care may be postponed until the medical examiner completes an investigation.

The write stuff

- Document the date and time of the patient's death and the name of the practitioner who pronounced the death.
- If resuscitation was attempted, indicate the time it started and ended, and refer to the code sheet in the patient's medical record.
- Note whether the case is being referred to the medical examiner.
- Include all postmortem care given, noting whether medical equipment was removed or left in place.
- List all belongings and valuables and the name of the family member who accepted and signed the appropriate valuables or belongings list.
- Record belongings left on the patient.
- If the patient has dentures, note whether they were left in the patient's mouth or given to a family member (if given to a family member, include the family member's name).

- Document the disposition of the patient's body and the name, telephone number, and address of the funeral home.
- List the names of family members who were present at the time of death.
- If the family wasn't present, note the name of the family member notified, the time he or she was notified, and who viewed the body.
- Include care, emotional support, and teaching given to the family.

08/22/06	1420	Called to room by pt.'s daughter, Mrs. Bridgitte
		Jones, stating pt. not breathing. Pt. found
		unresponsive in bed at 1345, not breathing, no
		pulse, no heart or breath sounds auscultated.
		No code called because pt. has advance
		directive and DNR order signed in chart. Case
		not referred to medical examiner. Death
		pronouncement made by Dr. Holmes at 1350.
		NG tube, Foley catheter, and I.V. line in Ⓛ
		forearm removed and dressings applied. Pt.
		bathed and given oral care, dentures placed in
		mouth, hair combed, and fresh linens and gown
		applied. Belongings checked off on belongings
		list and signed by Mrs. Jones, who will take
		belongings home with her. Pt. body tagged and
		sent to morgue at 1415. Mrs. Jones is making
		arrangements with Restful Funeral Home,
		123 Main St., Pleasantville, NY (123) 456-7890.
		Daughter states she's glad her dad isn't
		suffering any more. Stayed with daughter
		throughout her visit. Daughter stated she was
		OK to drive home. Declined visit by chaplain.
		Said she'll notify other family members who
		live out of state and won't be viewing body in
		hospital. ——————— Petra Gabriel, RN

Dehydration

- Dehydration, the loss of water in the body with a shift in fluid and electrolytes, can lead to hypovolemic shock, organ failure, and even death.
- Dehydration may be isotonic, hypertonic, or hypotonic.
- Common causes of dehydration are fever, diarrhea, and vomiting.
- Other causes include hemorrhage, excessive diaphoresis, burns, excessive wound or nasogastric drainage, and ketoacidosis.
- Prompt intervention is necessary to prevent complications.

The write stuff

- Record the date and time of your entry.
- Record the results of your physical assessment and subjective findings.
- Include laboratory values and the results of diagnostic tests.
- Record intake and output on an intake-output flow sheet.
- Record the name of the practitioner notified, the time of notification, and orders received.
- Document your interventions, such as I.V. therapy, and the patient's response.
- Record your actions to prevent complications, such as monitoring for I.V. infiltration and auscultating for breath sounds to detect fluid volume overload.
- Document patient teaching provided.

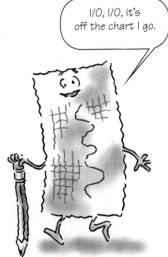

I/O, I/O, it's off the chart I go.

05/25/06	1345	Pt. admitted to unit from nursing home with
		increasing lethargy and diarrhea X3 days. Pt. is
		drowsy, doesn't answer questions, occasionally
		moans. Skin and mucous membranes dry;
		tenting occurs when pinched. P 118, BP 92/58,
		RR 28, rectal T 101.2° F, wt. 102 lb (family
		reports this is down 3 lb in 3 days). Breath
		sounds clear, normal heart sounds. Peripheral
		pulses palpable but weak. No edema. Dr. Holmes
		notified of assessment findings at 1315.
		Orders verbally accepted. Foley catheter
		inserted to monitor urine output. Urine
		sample sent to lab for UA and C&S. Urine
		color dark amber, specific gravity 1.001. Blood
		drawn for CBC with diff., BUN, creatinine, and
		electrolytes. Had approx. 300 ml of liquid
		stool, guaiac neg., sample sent for C&S. Dr.
		Holmes in to see pt. at 1330 and additional
		orders written. Pt. placed on cardiac monitor,
		no arrhythmias noted. Administering O_2 at 2L
		via NC. I.V. infusion started in Ⓛ upper
		forearm with 18G catheter. Infusing NSS at
		100 ml/hr. See I/O record and frequent vital
		signs assessment sheet for hourly VS and
		hourly I/O. ———— Claire Littleton, RN

Delayed transfusion reaction

- Transfusion reactions may occur 4 to 8 days or even up to 1 month after a blood transfusion.
- This type of reaction occurs in people who have developed antibodies from previous blood transfusions, which cause red blood cell hemolysis during subsequent transfusions.
- Reactions are typically mild and don't require treatment.
- If you suspect that a patient is having a delayed transfusion reaction, notify the practitioner and blood bank.
- Some facilities require you to complete a transfusion reaction report.

The write stuff

- Record the date and time of the suspected delayed transfusion reaction.
- Note the signs of a delayed reaction, such as fever, elevated white blood cell count, and a falling hematocrit.
- Record the name of the practitioner notified, the time of notification, orders received, and the time the practitioner came to see the patient.
- Include your interventions and the patient's response.
- Record the time that you notified the blood bank, the name of the person with whom you spoke, and orders received, such as obtaining blood or urine samples and sending them to the laboratory.
- Record patient teaching provided and the patient's reaction.

03/08/06	1215	Oral T 102.4° F at 1200. Pt. states he has
		chills, but no itching, nausea, or vomiting. No
		flushing, facial edema, or urticaria noted. P 82
		and regular, BP 128/72, RR 20 and unlabored.
		Lungs clear bilaterally. Labs from 0600 show
		hct 35%, hgb 12.4, WBC 15,000. Notified Dr.
		Green of elevated temp, assessment findings,
		and lab values at 1205. Dr. Green will see pt.
		at 1230. Notified Mike Cohen in blood bank of
		possible delayed transfusion reaction at 1210.
		Urine for UA and 2 red-top tubes of blood
		drawn and sent to lab. Explained to pt. that
		fever may be a possible delayed blood
		transfusion reaction and usually requires no
		treatment. —————————— Montgomery Burns, RN

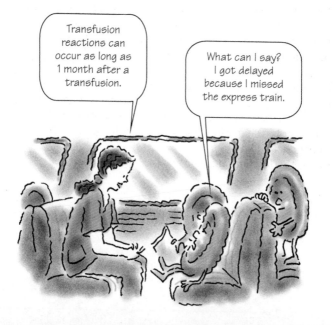

Transfusion reactions can occur as long as 1 month after a transfusion.

What can I say? I got delayed because I missed the express train.

Diagnostic testing

- Most patients undergo testing before receiving a diagnosis.
- Diagnostic testing may range from a simple blood test to a more complicated test such as magnetic resonance imaging.

The write stuff

- Document preliminary assessments you make of a patient's condition.
  - If the patient is pregnant or has certain allergies, record this information because it might affect the test or test result.
  - If the patient's age, illness, or disability requires special preparation for the test, enter this information in his chart.
- Document teaching you've done about the test and follow-up care associated with it.
- Include:
  - administration or withholding of drugs and preparations
  - special diets
  - food or fluid restrictions
  - enemas
  - specimen collection.

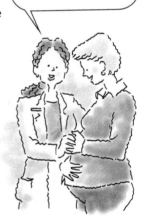

Document if the patient is pregnant because her condition may affect test results.

| 03/18/06 | 0700 | 24-hour urine test for creatinine clearance started. Pt. taught purpose of the test and how to collect urine. Pt. verbalized understanding of teaching and will collect his urine as instructed. Sign placed on pt.'s door and in bathroom. Urine placed on ice in bathroom. |
| | | ———————————————————— Charlie Pace, RN |

Discharge instructions

- Because hospitals discharge patients earlier than in years past, the patient and his family or caregiver must change dressings; assess wounds; deal with medical equipment, tube feedings, and I.V. lines; and perform other functions that a nurse traditionally performed.
- To perform these functions properly, you must provide the patient and his home caregiver with adequate instruction.
- If a patient receives improper instructions and injury results, you could be held liable.
- Many hospitals distribute printed instruction sheets that adequately describe treatments and home care procedures.
  - Courts typically consider these teaching materials evidence that instruction took place.
- Generally, the patient or responsible person must sign that he received and understood the discharge instructions.
- To support testimony that instructions were given, tailor written materials to each patient's specific needs and document verbal or written instructions that were provided.
- If caregivers practice procedures with the patient and family in the hospital, document their actions along with the results.
- Many facilities combine discharge summaries and patient instructions in one form, including sections for:
  - recording patient assessment
  - patient teaching
  - detailed special instructions
  - circumstances of discharge.

Form fitting

The discharge summary form

By combining the patient's discharge summary with instructions for care after discharge, you can fulfill two requirements with a single form. When using this documentation method, be sure to give one copy to the patient and keep one for the legal record.

DISCHARGE INSTRUCTIONS

1. Summary _Jackie Nicholas is a 55-year-old woman admitted with_
complaints of severe headache and hypertensive crisis.
    Treatment: Nitroprusside gtt for 24 hours
          Started Lopressor for hypertension
    Recommendation: Lose 10-15 lb
          Follow low-sodium, low-cholesterol diet

2. Allergies _penicillin — rash_

3. Medications (drug, dose time) _Lopressor 25 mg at 6 a.m. and 6 p.m._
    temazepam 15 mg at 10 p.m.

4. Diet _Low-sodium, low-cholesterol_

5. Activity _As tolerated_

6. Discharged to _Home_

7. If questions arise, contact Dr _Jack Shephard_
   Telephone No. _(233) 555-1448_

8. Special instructions _Call doctor with headaches, dizziness_

9. Return visit Dr. _Shephard_   Place _Health Care Clinic_
   On Date _12/15/06_   Time _0845 a.m._

Jackie Nicholas   _JE Shephard, MD_

Signature of patient or person responsible for receipt of instructions from doctors   Signature of doctor or nurse reviewing instructions

The write stuff

- Include the date and time of discharge.
- Note whether family members or caregivers were present for teaching.
- Document your teaching about treatments, such as dressing changes or use of medical equipment.
- Record signs and symptoms the patient is to report to the practitioner.
- Describe patient, family, or caregiver understanding of instructions or ability to give a return demonstration of procedures.
- Record whether a patient or caregiver requires further instruction.
- Include the practitioner's name and telephone number.
- Document that you told the patient the date, time, and location of follow-up appointments or that you informed him of the need to call the practitioner for a follow-up appointment.
- Give the details of instructions given to the patient, including those regarding medications, activity, and diet (include written instructions given to patient).
    - The patient's chart should indicate which materials were given and to whom.

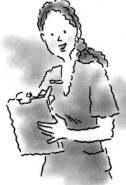

Record which patient teaching materials are given and to whom.

12/01/06	1530	Pt. to be discharged today. Reviewed discharge instructions with pt. and wife. Reviewed all medications, including drug name, purpose, doses, administration times, routes, and adverse effects. Drug information sheets given to pt. Pt. able to verbalize proper use of medications. Wife will be performing dressing change to pt.'s ⓛ foot. Wife was able to change dressing properly using sterile technique. Pt. and wife were able to state signs and symptoms of infections to report to doctor. Also reinforced low-cholesterol, low-sodium diet and progressive walking guidelines. Wife has many questions about diet and will meet with dietitian before discharge. Pt. understands he's to follow up with Dr. Carney in his office on 12/8/06 at 1400. Wrote doctor's phone number on written instructions. Written discharge instructions given to pt. ———Betty Davies, RN

Doctor's orders clarification

- Although unit secretaries may transcribe orders, the nurse is ultimately responsible for the accuracy of the transcription.
- Only you have the authority and knowledge to question the validity of orders and to spot errors.
- Follow your health care facility's policy for clarifying orders that are vague, ambiguous, or possibly erroneous.
- Contact the prescriber and document your actions.
- Delay treatment until you've contacted the prescriber and clarified the situation.

The write stuff

- Record your assessment and other data leading you to question the order.
- Include the name of the prescriber you notified and the time of notification.
- Document your conversation with the prescriber.
- Note whether the order was clarified or rewritten.
- Document whether the order was carried out and at what time.
- If you refuse to carry out an order you believe to be written in error, record your refusal, your reasons for refusing, the names of the prescriber and nursing supervisor you notified, the time of notification, and their responses.

| 09/07/06 | 1235 | Order written by Dr. Corrigan at 1155 for Darvocet N 1 tab P.O. q4hr prn incision pain. Called Dr. Corrigan at 1210 to clarify Darvocet dose. Order should read Darvocet-N 100 1 tablet P.O. q4hr prn incision pain. Clarification written on dr.'s orders and faxed to pharmacy. Dose changed on MAR. Darvocet N 100 given to pt. at 1220. ———— Meg Griffin, RN |

Do-not-resuscitate order

- When a patient is terminally ill and death is expected, the practitioner and family (and the patient if appropriate) may agree that a do-not-resuscitate (DNR), or no-code, order is appropriate.
- The practitioner writes the order, and the staff carries it out if the patient goes into cardiac or respiratory arrest.
- If a patient without a DNR order tells you he doesn't want to be resuscitated, follow your facility's policy and ask for assistance from administration, legal services, or social services.
- As a nurse, you have a responsibility to help the patient make an informed decision about continuing treatment.
- Because DNR orders are recognized legally, you'll incur no liability if you don't resuscitate a patient and that patient later dies; you may, however, incur liability if you initiate resuscitation on a patient who has a DNR order.
- Every patient with a DNR order should have a written order on file.
  – The order should be consistent with the facility's policy.
  – Policy commonly requires that DNR orders be reviewed every 48 to 72 hours.
- Health care facilities must provide written information to patients concerning their rights under state law to make decisions regarding their care.
  – Patients have the right to refuse medical treatment and the right to formulate an advance directive.
  – Information on advance directives must be provided upon admission.

The write stuff

- Document whether the patient has an advance directive and whether information about advance directives was given to him.

- If a terminally ill patient without a DNR order tells you that he doesn't want to be resuscitated in a crisis, document his:
  - statement (using his own words, in quotes, if possible)
  - degree of awareness and orientation.

> A patient's wishes may differ from those of his family. Include this information in the chart.

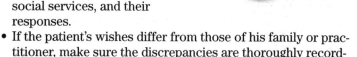

- Document the persons you contacted about the patient's wishes, such as the patient's practitioner, your nursing supervisor, legal services, or social services, and their responses.
- If the patient's wishes differ from those of his family or practitioner, make sure the discrepancies are thoroughly recorded in the chart.

06/19/06	1700	Pt. stated, "If my heart should stop or if I
		stop breathing, just let me go. I've suffered
		with this cancer long enough. I've lived a full
		life and have no regrets." Pt.'s wife was present
		for this conversation and stated, "I don't want
		to see him in pain anymore. If he feels he
		doesn't want any heroic measures, then I
		stand by his decision." Pt. is alert and oriented
		to time, place, and person. Dr. Patel notified
		of pt.'s wishes concerning resuscitation and
		stated he'll be in this evening to discuss DNR
		status with pt. and wife and write DNR orders.
		Elizabeth Sawyer, nursing supervisor, notified
		of pt.'s wishes for no resuscitation. ————
		———————————— Meryl Flynn, RN

Drug administration

- The medication administration record (MAR) is:
  - the central record of medication orders and their execution
  - part of the patient's permanent record
  - commonly included in a card file (a medication Kardex) or on a separate medication administration sheet.
- When administering drugs, know and follow your facility's policies and procedures for recording drug orders and charting drug administration.
- Document drugs using only standard abbreviations approved by your facility.
- Record drugs immediately after administration so that another nurse doesn't give the drug again.

The write stuff

- Record the patient's full name; the date; and the drug's name, dosage, administration route or method, and frequency on all drug orders.
- Include the specific number of doses given or stop date, when appropriate.
- Record drug allergy information.
- After administering the first dose, sign your full name, licensure status, and initials in the appropriate space on the MAR.

Keep me current! Chart each drug immediately after giving it.

- If you document by computer, chart your information for each drug immediately after you administer it, especially if you don't use printouts as a backup, so that all health care team members have access to the latest drug administration data for the patient.

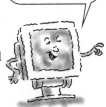

- If a specific assessment parameter must be monitored during administration of a drug, document this requirement on the MAR; for example, record the patient's apical pulse rate on the MAR when giving digoxin.

Form fitting

The medication Kardex

One type of Kardex is the medication Kardex. It contains a permanent record of the patient's medications. The medication Kardex may also include the patient's diagnosis and information about allergies and diet. Routine and p.r.n. drugs may be on separate forms. A sample form is shown below.

Name: _Jack Lemmons_   Medical record #: _1234567_

Nurse's full signature, status, and initials

	Init.		Init.		Init.
Roy Charles, RN	RC				
Theresa Hopkins, RN	TH				

Diagnosis: _Heart failure, atrial flutter, COPD_
Allergies: _ASA_   Diet: _Cardiac_

Routine/Daily orders			Date: 1/24/06		Date: 1/25/06		Date: 1/26/06		Date: 1/27/06		Date: 1/28/06	
Order Date	Medications: dose, route, frequency	Time	Site	Init.	Site	Init.	Site	Init.	Site	Init.	Site	Init.
1/24/06	digoxin 0.125 mg	0900	Ⓡ subclavian	RC		Ⓡ						
RC	I.V. daily	HR	68		52							
1/24/06	furosemide 40 mg	0900	Ⓡ subclavian	RC	Ⓡ subclavian	RC						
RC	I.V. q12hr	2100	Ⓡ subclavian	TH								
1/24/06	enalaprilat 1.25 mg	0500	Ⓡ subclavian	TH	Ⓡ subclavian	TH						
RC	I.V. q6hr	1100	Ⓡ subclavian	RC								
		1700	Ⓡ subclavian	RC								
		2300	Ⓡ subclavian	RC								

(continued)

The medication Kardex (continued)

PRN Medication

Addressograph   Allergies: ASA

Initial Signature and status   Initial Signature and status   Initial Signature and status

RC   Ray Charles, RN

TH   Theresia Hopkins, RN

Year 20 06   P.R.N. Medications

Order Renewal Discontinued					
Date: 1/24/06 Date: Date:	Date	1/24			
Medication: acetaminophen	Dose 650 mg	Time given	0930		
Direction p.r.n. mild pain	Route P.O.	Site	P.O.		
		Init.	RC		
Order Renewal Discontinued Date: 1/24/06 Date: 1/26/06 Date:	Date	1/24			
Medication: morphine sulfate	Dose 2 mg	Time given	0930		
Direction 15 min prior to changing ® heel dressing	Route I.V.	Site	® subclavian		
		Init.	RC		
Order Renewal Discontinued Date: 1/24/06 Date: Date:	Date	1/24			
Medication: Milk of Magnesia	Dose 30 ml	Time given	2115		
Direction q6hr p.r.n.	Route P.O.	Site	P.O.		
		Init.	TH		
Order Renewal Discontinued Date: 1/25/06 Date: Date: 1/25/06	Date	1/25	1/25		
Medication: prochlorperazine	Dose 5 mg	Time given	1100	2230	
Direction q8hr p.r.n.	Route P.O.	Site	P.O.	P.O.	
		Init.	RC	TH	
Order Renewal Discontinued Date: 1/25/06 Date: Date: 1/25/06	Date	1/25			
Medication: fluzone	Dose 0.5 ml	Time given	1100		
Direction Give 1 dose only	Route I.M.	Site	® delt.		
		Init.	RC		
Order Renewal Discontinued Date: 1/25/06 Date: Date: 1/25/06	Date	1/25			
Medication: furosemide	Dose 40 mg	Time given	1300		
Direction stat now	Route I.V.	Site	® subclavian		
		Init.	RC		

Drug overdose

- An overdose is consumption of drugs in an amount that produces a life-threatening response.
- Overdose can be intentional (such as a suicide gesture or attempt) or accidental (such as overmedicating with pain medicine).
- If you suspect a drug overdose, immediately contact a practitioner and take measures to ensure the patient's airway, breathing, and circulation.
- Other interventions focus on identifying, removing, and neutralizing the drug as well as enhancing its excretion.

The write stuff

- Record the date and time of your entry.
- Chart a brief medical history, if possible, including:
  - allergies
  - current drugs
  - history of substance abuse.
- Record:
  - type and amount of drug taken
  - route of ingestion
  - signs and symptoms exhibited.
- Document vital signs, noting the character of respirations and strength of pulses.
- Note the patient's mental status, including level of consciousness, orientation, and ability to follow commands.
- Document your neurologic assessment, including:
  - pupillary reaction
  - cranial nerve assessment
  - fine and gross motor activity
  - sensory functioning
  - reflexes.
- Record the findings of your cardiopulmonary assessment.
- If appropriate, record interventions implemented before the patient's arrival at your facility.

- Note the name of the practitioner notified, time of notification, and orders received.
- Document your interventions, such as administering reversal agents (naloxone [Narcan] and flumazenil [Romazicon]) or GI decontaminants (activated charcoal, ipecac syrup, gastric lavage, cathartics, and whole-bowel irrigation), as well as supportive therapies. Include the patient's response.
- If gastric emptying is performed, document the character and contents of the emesis.
- Use flow sheets to record your frequent assessments, vital signs, intake and output, I.V. therapy, and laboratory values.
- Record your patient teaching, including strategies to prevent future drug overdose.
- Document emotional support given.

09/17/06	0200	Pt. admitted to ED at 0140 with suspected opioid overdose. EMTs said a friend of the pt.'s at the scene said the pt. may have taken "pain killers." Lab called for stat toxicology screen, CBC, BUN, creatinine, electrolytes, and ABGs. Pt. unresponsive to painful stimulation. HR 56, BP 100/50, tympanic T 96.8° F. Pupils pinpoint and nonreactive to light. Muscle tone in extremities flaccid, deep tendon reflexes absent. Pt. was intubated in the field and is receiving rescue breathing via AMBU with 100% FIO_2. Bilateral chest expansion present and breath sounds clear. Dr. Weaver called at 0145 and orders received. I.V. access established in ℞ antecubital vein with 18G catheter. 1000 ml NSS infusing at 100 ml/hr. Naloxone I.V. push administered. See MAR. Pt. immediately began moving extremities and coughing. Attempted to remove ET tube. He was calmed and instructed regarding treatment. He nodded his head to acknowledge understanding instructions. See flow sheets for frequent VS, I/O, I.V. therapy, and labs. ———————— James Ford, RN

Drug refusal

- If a patient refuses to take his prescribed drugs, notify his practitioner and describe the event in his chart.
- By documenting the refusal, you avoid the misinterpretation that you omitted the drug by mistake.

The write stuff

- Record the date and time of your entry.
- Document that your patient refused to take his prescribed drugs and the reason, using his own words in quotes, if possible.
- Record the name of the refused drugs and the time they were due.
- Include explanations given on the indications for the drugs and why they were ordered for the patient.
- Note the name of the practitioner notified, the time of notification, and orders received.

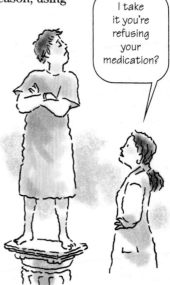

I take it you're refusing your medication?

02/05/06	1015	Pt. refused K-Dur tabs scheduled for 1000, stating that they were "too big to swallow." Dr. Morris notified at 1005. K-Dur tabs discontinued. KCL elixir ordered and given. ———— Carrie Bradshaw, RN

Dyspnea

- Dyspnea is the sensation of difficult or uncomfortable breathing.
  - Usually, it's reported as shortness of breath.
  - It's commonly a symptom of cardiopulmonary dysfunction.
- Dyspnea may arise suddenly or slowly and may subside rapidly or persist for years.
  - Most people experience dyspnea when they overexert themselves.
  - Its severity depends on the patient's physical condition; in the healthy person, dyspnea is quickly relieved by rest.
- Causes include pulmonary, cardiac, neuromuscular, and allergic disorders and anxiety.
- Whatever the cause of dyspnea, place the patient in an upright position, unless contraindicated, and perform a rapid respiratory assessment.
- Prepare to administer oxygen by nasal cannula, mask, or endotracheal tube.
- Start an I.V. infusion and begin cardiac monitoring to detect arrhythmias.
- Anticipate interventions, such as inserting a chest tube for pneumothorax, giving a morphine injection to treat pulmonary edema, or administering breathing treatments for acute asthma.

The write stuff

- Record the date and time of your entry.
- State the problem in the patient's own words, if he can communicate.
- If it's appropriate, ask these questions and document the patient's responses:
  - What was he doing when the dyspnea started?
  - Did it begin gradually or suddenly?
  - Does it occur at rest or with activity?

- What aggravates or alleviates the dyspnea?
- Does he have a productive or nonproductive cough?
- Does he have a history of recent trauma or disease?
- Does he smoke?
- Does he have accompanying symptoms, such as orthopnea, paroxysmal nocturnal dyspnea, or progressive fatigue?

• Document your cardiopulmonary examination, including:
  - vital signs
  - respiratory rate, depth, and effort
  - breath and heart sounds
  - use of accessory muscles
  - skin color
  - presence of edema
  - mental status
  - chest pain.
• Record the name of the practitioner notified, the time of notification, and orders received.
• Include diagnostic tests and results, if available, such as chest X-ray, pulse oximetry, arterial blood gas analysis, hemoglobin level, hematocrit, pulmonary function tests, and electrocardiography.
• Describe your interventions and their results, such as cardiac monitoring, administering oxygen, I.V. infusions, medications, breathing treatments, and positioning.
• Document patient teaching, such as how to perform coughing and deep breathing, pursed-lip breathing, relaxation techniques, and incentive spirometry.
• Include emotional support given.

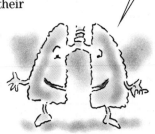

I suggest you make it your quest to document diagnostic tests such as X-rays to the chest.

01/03/06	0900	Pt. c/o SOB after walking from bathroom to bed, approx. 25'. Assisted pt. back to bed, placed him in high Fowler's position, re-attached to O_2 at 2 L/min by NC. Lungs with scattered rhonchi, bilaterally. P 118, BP 132/90, RR 40 labored with use of accessory muscles, axillary T 97.4° F, O_2 sat. by pulse oximetry 87%. Heart sounds within normal limits. Skin pale, +1 edema of both ankles. Pt. alert and oriented to time, place, and person. No c/o chest pain. Pt. stated "I haven't been moving around much at home because it's getting harder and harder to breathe." He said he's been discussing the use of O_2 at home with his doctor. Dr. Smith notified at 0850 and came to see pt. Ordered O_2 to be used when out of bed and ambulating. Carla Moore, in respiratory therapy, notified. Pt. instructed to cough and deep-breathe q1hr while awake. Coughed up moderate amount of white sputum. ———————— ———————————————— San Kwon, RN
01/03/06	0920	Pt. states he's no longer SOB. P 102, BP 130/88, RR 20, with less effort. Not using accessory muscles. O_2 sat. by pulse oximetry 97%. Main-taining O_2 at 2 L/min by NC. —— San Kwon, RN

Elopement

- Elopement is when a patient is missing or has left the health care facility without having said anything about leaving.
- When you discover a patient is missing, immediately look for him on your unit and notify the nurse manager, security, the patient's practitioner, and the patient's family.
- Notify the police if the patient is at risk for harming himself or others.
- The legal consequences of a patient leaving the facility without medical permission can be particularly severe, especially if he's confused, mentally incompetent, or injured or if he dies of exposure as a result of his absence.

The write stuff

- Document the time that you discovered the patient missing.
- Describe your attempts to find the patient.
- Record the names of the people you notified.

03/25/06	0800	Entered pt.'s room to administer his medication
		and discovered pt. wasn't in his room. Pt.'s
		bathroom and unit were searched. Hospital
		security; Beth Welsh, nurse-manager; and
		Dr. Kovac notified. Pt.'s family called and
		informed that he was missing. ————————
		—————————————————— Elona Levine, RN

Endotracheal extubation

- When your patient no longer requires endotracheal (ET) intubation, the airway can be removed according to facility
  policy.
- When performing the procedure:
  - explain the procedure to the patient
  - obtain another nurse's assistance to prevent traumatic ma-
    nipulation of the tube when it's untaped or unfastened.
- Teach the patient to cough and deep-breathe after the ET
  tube is removed.
- Assess the patient frequently for signs of respiratory distress.

The write stuff

- Record the date and time of extubation.
- Note the presence or absence of stridor or other signs of upper airway edema.
- Document if suctioning was required before extubation and include a description
  of secretions.
- Record who extubated the patient and the
  time the procedure was performed.
- Document the patient's breath sounds.
- Chart the type of sup-
  plemental oxygen ad-
  ministered.
- Note complications
  and required subse-
  quent therapy.

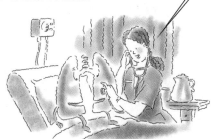

Your breath sounds are top of the charts!

- Note the patient's tolerance of the procedure and subsequent therapy.
- Document patient teaching and support given.

05/26/06	1700	Explained extubation procedure to pt. Pt. acknowledged understanding by nodding his head "yes." Placed pt. in high Fowler's position and suctioned for scant amount of thin white secretions. ET tube removed at 1630. No stridor or respiratory distress noted, breath sounds clear. RR 22, P 92, BP 128/82, oral T 98.4° F. Pulse oximetry 97% on O₂ 2 L by NC. Pt. states he's happy to have tube out. Instructed pt. on importance of coughing and deep breathing every hr. Pt. was able to give proper return demonstration. Cough nonproductive. ———— _Margie Simpson, RN_

Endotracheal intubation

- Endotracheal (ET) intubation involves the oral or nasal insertion of a flexible tube through the larynx into the trachea for the purposes of:
  - establishing and maintaining a patent airway
  - protecting against aspiration by sealing off the trachea from the digestive tract
  - permitting removal of tracheobronchial secretions in patients who can't cough effectively
  - providing a route for mechanical ventilation.
- The procedure is performed according to facility policy by a practitioner, anesthetist, respiratory therapist, or nurse educated in the procedure.
- ET intubation usually occurs in emergencies, such as cardiopulmonary arrest or respiratory distress, or diseases, such as epiglottitis, but it may also occur in controlled circumstances; for example, just before surgery.
- ET intubation requires patient teaching and preparation.

The write stuff

- Document that the practitioner explained the procedure, risks, complications, and alternatives to the patient or person responsible for making decisions concerning the patient's health care.
- Indicate that the patient or health care proxy consented to the procedure.
- Record the date and time of intubation and the name of the person performing the procedure.
- Include indications for the procedure and whether the procedure was successful.

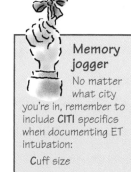

Memory jogger
No matter what city you're in, remember to include **CITI** specifics when documenting ET intubation:

Cuff size
Inflation amount
Tube size
Inflation technique.

- Chart the type and size of tube, cuff size, amount of inflation, and inflation technique.
- Indicate whether drugs were administered.
- Document the initiation of supplemental oxygen or ventilation therapy.
- Record the results of chest auscultation and chest X-ray.
- Note the occurrence of complications, necessary interventions, and the patient's response.
- Describe the patient's reaction to the procedure.
- Document teaching done before and after the procedure.

| 03/16/06 | 1015 | Pt. informed by Dr. Eagan of the need for intubation, the risks, potential complications, and alternatives. Pt. consented to the procedure. Pt. given midazolam 5 mg by I.V. and intubated by Dr. Langley at 0945 with size 8 oral cuffed ET tube. Tube taped in place in right corner of mouth. Cuff inflated with 5 ml of air. Pt. on ventilator set at TV 750, FIO_2 45%, 5 cm PEEP, AC of 12. RR 20, nonlabored. Portable CXR confirms proper placement. ® lung with basilar crackles and expiratory wheezes. Ⓛ lung clear. Pt. opening eyes when name is called. When asked if he's comfortable and in no pain, pt. nods head "yes." ———————— Dom Hanks, RN |

Endotracheal tube removal by patient

- Because an endotracheal (ET) tube is used to provide mechanical ventilation and maintain a patent airway, the removal of an ET tube by a patient is an emergency situation.
- The patient may not have spontaneous respirations, may be in severe respiratory distress, or may suffer trauma to the larynx or vocal cords.
- If your patient removes his ET tube:
  - Stay with him and call for help.
  - Assign someone to notify the practitioner while you assess the patient's respiratory status.
  - If the patient is in distress, perform manual ventilation while others prepare for reinsertion of the ET tube and monitor vital signs.
  - If your patient is alert, speak calmly and explain the reintubation procedure.
  - If the patient isn't in distress, provide oxygen therapy.
  - If the decision is made not to reintubate the patient, monitor his respiratory status and vital signs every 15 minutes for 2 to 3 hours, or as ordered.

The write stuff

- Record the date and time of your entry.
- Note how you discovered the ET tube was removed by the patient.
- Record your respiratory assessment.
- Record the name of the practitioner notified and the time of notification.
- Document your actions, such as oxygen therapy and manual ventilation, and the patient's response.
- If the patient required reinsertion of the ET tube, follow the procedure for documenting ET intubation.
- Record patient teaching and emotional support provided.

01/30/06	0400	Summoned to room by ventilator alarms at
		0330. Found pt. in bed with ET tube in hand.
		P 86 and regular, BP 140/70, RR 32 regular
		and deep. No use of accessory muscles, skin
		warm, dry, and pink, O_2 sat. by pulse oximetry
		94%. Lungs clear to auscultation bilaterally. Pt.
		oriented to time, place, and person. Pt. stated
		in a raspy voice, "I must have been dreaming.
		And when I woke up, the tube was in my hand."
		Administered O_2 at 4 L by NC with O_2 sat.
		97%. Stayed with pt. while another nurse
		notified Dr. Smith at 0335. Dr. Smith came
		to see pt. at 0345 and, after assessing pt.,
		made decision to keep ET tube out. Plan is
		to maintain O_2 at 4 L by NC and monitor
		pt.'s respiratory status q 15 min for 2 hr.
		Instructed pt. on the use of incentive
		spirometer q1hr while awake. Pt. was able to
		give proper return demonstration and
		verbalized understanding that it should be
		performed every hour. ——— Michael Dawson, RN

Enema administration

- An enema is a solution introduced into the rectum and colon.
- Enemas are used to:
  - administer medication
  - clean the lower bowel in preparation for diagnostic or surgical procedures
  - relieve distention and promote expulsion of flatus
  - lubricate the rectum and colon
  - soften hardened stool for removal.
- Enema solutions and methods vary to suit your patient's condition or treatment requirements.

The write stuff

- Record the time the practitioner was notified of the patient's complaint of constipation and that an order for an enema was given.
- Record the date and time of enema administration.
- Include the type of enema given, such as cleansing, lubricating, or carminative, and the procedure used to instill the enema.
- Write down the type and amount of solution used, the retention time, and approximate amount returned.
- Describe the color, consistency, and amount of the return, and any abnormalities with the return.
- Record complications that occurred, actions taken, and the patient's response.

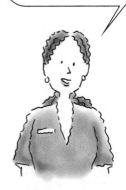

Check your facility's policy to determine if an enema needs to be documented on the medication Kardex.

- Document the patient's tolerance of the procedure.
- Depending on your facility's policy, you may also need to document the enema on the medication Kardex or treatment record.

| 02/28/06 | 0900 | Pt. c/o constipation. States she hasn't had a BM for 2 days. Dr. Pratt notified at 0815 and ordered Fleet enema 1 daily p.r.n. constipation. Procedure, risks, and alternatives explained to pt. and she consented. Fleet enema, 100 ml, given to pt. at 0830 and held for 20 minutes. Pt. had large amount of brown, solid stool. No c/o abd. pain; no abd. distention noted. ——————————————— Francie Sinatra, R.N |

Epidural analgesia

- With epidural analgesia, an epidural catheter is placed by an anesthesiologist in the epidural space outside the spinal cord between the vertebrae.
- A local anesthetic—either alone or in combination with an opioid, such as preservative-free morphine or fentanyl—is administered through the catheter and moves slowly into the cerebrospinal fluid to opiate receptors in the dorsal horn of the spinal cord.
- Drug delivery so close to the opiate receptors provides pain relief with minimal adverse effects.
- Opioids may be administered:
  - by bolus dose, continuous infusion by pump, or patient-controlled analgesia.
  - alone or in combination with bupivacaine (a local anesthetic).
- Monitor the patient for these adverse reactions and notify the practitioner or anesthesiologist if they occur:
  - sedation
  - nausea
  - urinary retention
  - orthostatic hypotension
  - itching
  - respiratory depression
  - headache
  - back soreness
  - leg weakness and numbness.
- Most facilities have policies that address interventions for adverse effects and monitoring parameters.
- Monitor the patient frequently for the first 12 hours, and then every 4 hours after that, according to facility policy.

- Most facilities use a flow sheet to document:
  - drug dosage, rate, route
  - vital signs
  - respiratory rate
  - pulse oximetry
  - pain scale
  - sedation scale.
- If you don't have a specific flow sheet for epidural documentation, use your regular flow sheet and document in the progress notes other assessments or unusual circumstances as needed.

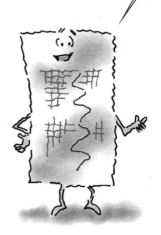

Your facility may have a specific flow sheet for epidural documentation.

The write stuff

- Record the date and time of your entry.
- Document the type and dose of the drug administered.
- Include the patient's:
  - level of consciousness
  - pain level (using a 0-to-10 scale, with 0 being no pain and 10 being the worst pain imaginable)
  - respiratory rate and quality.
- Record the amount of drug received per hour and the number of dose attempts by the patient if the analgesia is patient-controlled.
- Chart your assessment of the site, dressing changes, infusion bag changes, tubing changes, and patient teaching.
- Document complications, such as numbness, leg weakness, and respiratory depression, your interventions, and the patient's response.

05/22/06	0500	Pt. received from PACU with epidural catheter
		in place. Dressing covering site clean, dry, and
		intact. Pt. receiving bupivacaine 0.125% and
		fentanyl 5 mcg/ml in 250 ml NSS at rate of
		2 ml/hr. Respiratory rate 20 and deep, level
		of sedation 0 (alert), O_2 sat. by pulse oximetry
		on O_2 2L by NC 99%, BP 120/80, P 72. Pt.
		reports pain as 2 on a scale of 0 to 10, w/10
		being worst pain imaginable. No c/o nausea,
		itching, H/A, leg weakness, back soreness. Pt.
		voided 300 ml yellow urine. Bladder scan
		shows no residual after void. Told pt. to
		report any pain greater than 3 out of 10,
		inability to void, and numbness in legs. Epidural
		infusion label applied to catheter, infusion
		tubing, and infusion pump. See flow sheet for
		frequent monitoring of drug dose, rate, VS,
		resp. rate, pulse ox., level of pain, and
		sedation level. ———————— Tara Brown, RN

Evidence collection

- You may be asked by the police to collect evidence from an injured suspect in your care.
  - For example, they may ask you to give them the patient's belongings and a sample of his blood.
- If you fail to follow proper protocol, the evidence you turn over to the police may not be admissible in court or the patient may sue you for invasion of privacy.
- If an accused person consents to a search, all evidence found is considered admissible in court.
- Opinions differ as to whether a blood test, such as an alcohol blood test, is admissible in court if the person refused consent for the test.
- A nurse who does blood work without the patient's consent may be liable for committing battery, even if the patient is a suspected criminal and the blood work is medically necessary.
- Consult an administrator or hospital attorney before complying with a police request to turn over a patient's personal property.
- Until evidence can be turned over to the police, it should be kept in a locked area.

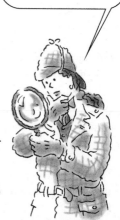

Whether you use a specific chain of custody form or detailed notes, keep track of what evidence was taken, who took it, and when.

The write stuff

- Note blood work done.
- List all treatments and the patient's response to them.
- Record anything you turn over to the police or administration and the name of the person you gave it to.

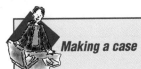

Making a case

To search or not to search?

The Fourth Amendment to the U.S. Constitution provides that "the right of the people to be secure in their persons, houses, papers, and effects, against unreasonable searches and seizures shall not be violated, and no warrants shall be issued, but upon probable cause." This means that every individual, even a suspected criminal, has a right to privacy, including a right to be free from intrusions that are made without search warrants. However, the Fourth Amendment doesn't absolutely prohibit all searches and seizures, only the unreasonable ones.

Respect rights
In general, searches that occur as part of medical care don't violate a suspect's rights. However, searches made for the sole purpose of gathering evidence — especially if done at police request — may. Several courts have said that a suspect subjected to an illegal private search has a right to seek remedy against the unlawful searcher in a civil lawsuit.

Always check
Because the laws of search and seizure are complex and subject to change by new legal decisions, consult an administrator or hospital attorney before complying with a police request to turn over a patient's personal propoerty.

- Statements made by the patient should be recorded only if they're directly related to his care.
- Document the presence of a police officer and your interactions with the officer.
- Document the name of the administrator or hospital attorney you consulted before turning anything over to the police.

- If you discover evidence, use your facility's chain of custody form to document the identity of each person handling the evidence as well as the dates and times it was in each person's possession.
- If your facility doesn't have a chain of custody form:
  - Keep detailed notes of exactly what was taken, by whom, and when.
  - Give this information to the administrator when you deliver the evidence.

| 12/02/06 | 2120 | Mr. Piper was escorted by a police officer to the ED at 2045 with four lacerations on Ⓛ leg. Pt. smelled of alcohol and cigarette smoke. He was calm but easily agitated. While cutting his pant leg to remove his pants, a ziplock bag with a white powder fell to the floor. In addition, a pocketknife, $6.87, and a pen were collected. Officer Smitts requested the knife and bag of white powder. After discussing the request with Arnold Becker, Chief Administrator, the knife and bag of powder were turned over to Officer Smitts. The remaining items and clothing, which consisted of pen, brown belt, and lightweight blue jacket, were bagged and left with pt. Pt. states he had tetanus shot last year. Lacerations of Ⓛ leg were irrigated with sterile NSS, stitched by Dr. Lewis after administering local anesthetic injections, antibiotic ointment applied, and covered with dry sterile dressings. Mr. Piper reports only minimal discomfort at laceration site. Explained care of lacerations and signs and symptoms of infection to report. Pt. verbalized understanding. Written ED guidelines for care of stitches given to pt. ———— Sam Taggart, RN |

F

Falls

- Falls are a major cause of injury and death among elderly people.
- In acute care hospitals:
  - 85% of all inpatient incident reports are related to falls.
  - 10% of people who fall do so more than once and 10% experience a fatal fall.
- In nursing homes, about 60% of residents fall every year and 40% of those residents experience more than one fall.
- If your patient falls:
  - Stay with him.
  - Don't move him until you've performed a head-to-toe assessment and checked his vital signs.
  - Assign another person to notify the practitioner.
  - Provide emergency measures necessary, such as securing an airway, controlling bleeding, or stabilizing a deformed limb.
  - If you don't detect problems, return the patient to bed with the help of another person.
  - File an incident report and chart the event.
  - Be objective in your documentation, avoiding judgments or opinions.

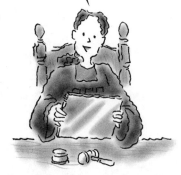

I'm allowed to be judgmental. Your documentation isn't. Be objective.

The write stuff

- Record how the patient was found and the time he was discovered.
- Ask the patient or witness what happened and document the response using his own words, in quotes, if possible.
- Include emergency interventions and the patient's response.
- Ask the patient if he's in pain or hit his head, and document his response.
- Chart the results of your head-to-toe assessment.
- Record bruises, lacerations, or abrasions.
- Describe pain or deformity in the extremities, particularly the hip, arm, leg, or lumbar spine.
- Record vital signs, including orthostatic blood pressure.
- Document your patient's neurologic assessment, noting slurred speech, weakness in the extremities, or a change in mental status.
- Record the name of the practitioner and other persons notified, such as the nursing supervisor or family members, and the time of notification.
- Include instructions or orders received.
- Document patient teaching given.

11/06/06	1400	Pt. found on floor between bed and chair on left side of bed at 1330. Pt. c/o pain in her ® hip area and difficulty moving ® leg. No abrasions or lacerations noted. BP elevated at 158/94. Didn't move pt. to determine ortho-static changes, P 94, RR 22, oral T 98.2° F. Pt states, "I was trying to get into the chair when I fell." Pt. alert and oriented to time, place, and person. Speech clear and coherent. Hand grasps strong bilaterally. ® leg externally rotated and shorter than Ⓛ leg. Dr. Jarrah notified at 1338. Pt. assisted back to bed with assist of 3, maintaining ® hip and leg in alignment. Hip X-ray ordered and showed ® hip fracture. Dr. Jarrah aware and family notified. Pt. to be evaluated by orthopedic surgeon. Pt. medicated for pain with Demerol 50 mg I.M. Maintaining bed rest at present time. Explaining all procedures to pt. Call bell in hand and understands to call for help with moving. ——————————— Jamie Stewart, RN

Fall precautions

- Patient falls resulting from slips, slides, knees giving way, fainting, or tripping over equipment can lead to prolonged hospitalization, increased hospital costs, and liability problems.
- Your facility may require you to assess each patient for his risk of falling and to take measures to prevent falls.
- If your facility requires a risk assessment form for patients, complete it and keep it in the patient's chart.
- Those at risk require a care plan reflecting interventions to prevent falls.

The write stuff

- Record the time and date of your entry.
- Describe the reasons for implementing fall precautions for your patient, such as a high score on a risk for falls assessment tool.

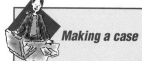

Making a case

Reducing your liability in patient falls

Patient falls are a very common area of nursing liability. Patients who are elderly, infirm, sedated, or mentally incapacitated are the most likely to fall. The case of *Stevenson v. Alta Bates* (1937) involved a patient who had a stroke and was learning to walk again. As two nurses, each holding one of the patient's arms, assisted her into the hospital's sunroom, one of the nurses let go of the patient and stepped forward to get a chair for her. The patient fell and sustained a fracture. The nurse was found negligent: The court said she should have anticipated the patient's need for a chair and made the appropriate arrangements before bringing the patient into the sunroom.

- Document interventions, such as:
  - frequent toileting
  - reorienting the patient to his environment
  - placing needed objects within the patient's reach.
- Include the patient's response to these interventions.
- Note measures taken to alert other health care workers of the risk for falls, such as placing a band on the patient's wrist and communicating this risk on the patient's Kardex.
- Record patient and family teaching given and their level of understanding.

01/26/06	1000	Score of 13 on admission Risk Assessment for Falls form. High risk for falls communicated to pt. and family. Risk for falls ID placed on pt.'s L wrist, high-risk for falls checked off on care plan and Kardex. Pt. alert and oriented to time, place, and person. Oriented pt. and family to room and call bell system. Told pt. to call for help before getting out of bed or up from chair on his own. Pt. demonstrated proper use of call bell and verbalized when to use it. Personal items and call bell placed within reach. ——————— *Betty Grabled, RN*

Form fitting

Risk assessment for falls

To use this risk assessment for falls form, check each applicable item and total the number of points. A score of 10 or more indicates a risk of falling.

DETERMINING A PATIENT'S RISK OF FALLING

Patient name: *John Fallen* **Medical record #:** *911911*

Pts.   Patient category

Age
1 ☐ 80 or older
2 ☑ 70 to 79 years old

Mental state
0 ☐ Oriented at all times or comatose
2 ☐ Confused at all times
4 ☑ Confused periodically

Duration of hospitalization
0 ☑ Over 3 days
2 ☐ 0 to 3 days

Falls within the past 6 months
0 ☐ None
2 ☑ 1 or 2
5 ☐ 3 or more

Elimination
0 ☑ Independent and continent
1 ☐ Uses catheter, ostomy, or both
3 ☐ Needs help with elimination
5 ☐ Independent and incontinent

1 ☑ *Visual impairment*

3 ☐ *Confinement to chair*

Pts.   Patient category

2 ☐ *Blood pressure*
Drop in systolic pressure of 20 mm Hg or more between lying and standing positions

Gait and balance
Assess gait by having the patient stand in one spot with both feet on the ground for 30 seconds without holding onto something. Then have him walk straight ahead and through a doorway. Next, have him turn while walking.
1 ☐ Wide base of support
1 ☐ Loss of balance while standing
1 ☑ Balance problems when walking
1 ☐ Diminished muscle coordination
1 ☐ Lurching or swaying
1 ☐ Holds on or changes gait when walking through a doorway
1 ☐ Jerking or instability when turning
1 ☐ Needs an assistive device such as a walker

(continued)

Risk assessment for falls *(continued)*

Pts. **Patient category**
Medications
How many different drugs is the patient taking?
0 ☐ None
1 ☐ 1
2 ☑ 2 or more

☐ Alcohol   ☐ Antidiabetics   ☐ Psychotropics
☐ Anesthetics   ☑ Benzodiazepines   ☐ Sedative-hypnotics
☐ Antihistamines   ☐ Cathartics   ☐ Other drugs (specify)
☑ Antihypertensives   ☐ Diuretics   _____
☐ Antiseizure drugs   ☐ Opioids   _____

1 ☑ Check if the patient has changed drugs, dosage, or both in the past 5 days.

<u>13</u>   TOTAL

Date/Time: _9/15/07 1300_   **Signature:** _Harriet Rachet, RN_

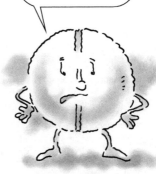

Numerous factors, such as age, mental status, and medication use, can increase your patient's risk of falling.

Family questions about care

- The family of a patient may have questions about the quality of care that a family member is receiving.
- Concerns should be taken seriously—ignoring them increases the risk of a lawsuit.
- Don't argue with the family, and avoid defending yourself, a coworker, a practitioner, or the facility.
- When family members question the quality of care:
  - show that you're concerned
  - ask them to clarify what they believe to be the problem.
- Provide teaching about nursing routines, policies, procedures and, within the limits of confidentiality, the patient's care plan.
- If the concern isn't a nursing issue:
  - Help the family find the answers to their questions.
  - Ask the practitioner, nursing supervisor, or another appropriate person to speak with the family.
- Report all unresolved concerns about the quality of care to your nursing supervisor or risk manager.

The write stuff

- Record the date and time of your conversation with the family.
- Include the names of the family members present.
- Document the concerns using their own words, in quotes, if possible.

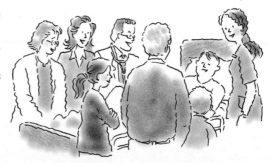

Families matter. Take their questions seriously.

- Describe your answers and the family members' responses.
- Record the names of the people you notified of the family's concerns, including the practitioner, nursing supervisor, and risk manager, and the time of notification.
- Document your conversation and their responses in quotes.

06/22/06	1600	Pt.'s daughter, Emily Jones, verbalized concerns regarding mother's hygiene. She stated, "I don't think my mother is receiving her showers. Her hair and fingernails are dirty." After reviewing the shower schedule, explained to Mrs. Jones that her mother has been refusing 1 of her 2 scheduled showers each week since admission 2 weeks ago and has been receiving sponge baths instead. Nurses' notes indicate that pt. stated, "I've never taken more than 1 shower per week in my entire life and I don't intend to start now." Records also show that for the last 2 days pt. has been participating in planting flower boxes around the facility. Mrs. Jones spoke with her mother and reported that "my mother will continue to shower once per week, sponge bathe on a daily basis, and have an appointment at the facility beauty salon once per week." Care plan amended to reflect this. —————— Liz Barton, RN

G

Gastric lavage

- After poisoning or a drug overdose, especially in patients who have central nervous system depression or an inadequate gag reflex, gastric lavage is used to flush the stomach and remove ingested substances through a gastric lavage tube.
- For patients with gastric or esophageal bleeding, a lavage with normal saline solution may be used to stop bleeding.
- Gastric lavage is contraindicated after ingestion of a corrosive substance, such as lye, ammonia, or mineral acids, because the lavage tube may perforate the already compromised esophagus.
- Typically, a doctor, gastroenterologist, or nurse performs this procedure in the emergency department or intensive care unit.
- Correct lavage tube placement is essential for patient safety because accidental misplacement (in the lungs, for example) followed by lavage can be fatal.

The write stuff

- If possible, note:
  - type of substance ingested
  - when the ingestion occurred
  - how much substance was ingested.
- Record preprocedure vital signs and level of consciousness (LOC).
- Record:
  - the date and time of lavage
  - size and type of nasogastric tube used
  - volume and type of irrigant
  - amount of drained gastric contents, including the color and consistency of drainage.

- Document the amount of irrigant solution instilled and gastric contents drained on the intake and output record sheet.
- Note whether drainage was sent to the laboratory for analysis.
- Record drugs instilled through the tube.
- Chart vital signs every 15 minutes on a frequent vital signs assessment sheet and LOC on a Glasgow Coma Scale sheet until the patient is stable.
- Indicate the time that the tube was removed and how the patient tolerated the procedure.

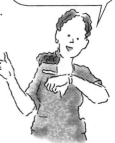

After gastric lavage, you'll need to chart vital signs every 15 minutes until the patient is stable.

| 04/22/06 | 2300 | Single lumen #30 Fr. Ewald tube placed by Dr. Reyes at 2230, without difficulty, for gastric lavage following ingestion of unknown quantity of diazepam. Prelavage P 56, BP 90/52, RR 14 and shallow, rectal T 97.0° F. Pt. lethargic, unresponsive to verbal stimuli, but responsive to painful stimuli, gag reflex present but diminished, reflexes hypoactive, PEARLA. Lavage performed with 250 ml NSS, returned contents liquid green with small blue flecks and some undigested food. Sample collected and sent to lab for analysis. Postprocedure P 58, BP 90/54, RR 15, LOC unchanged. ———————————— Erin Presley, RN |
| 04/22/06 | 2315 | Lavage repeated x2 with 500 ml NSS each. Gastric return clear after third lavage. Total return 1375 ml. P 60, BP 94/52, RR 15. Lethargic but responsive to verbal stimuli, reflexes still sluggish. q15min VS and LOC documented on frequent vital signs and Glasgow Coma Scale sheets. Gastric tube left in place until pt. alert. ——— Erin Presley, RN |

Gastrointestinal hemorrhage

- GI hemorrhage is the loss of a large amount of blood from the GI tract.
- Bleeding in the upper GI tract is caused primarily by ulcers, varices, or tears within the GI system.
- Lower GI bleeding may be caused by diverticulitis, polyps, ulcerative colitis, or cancer.
- Immediate lifesaving interventions focus on stabilizing the cardiovascular system, identifying the bleeding source, and stopping the bleeding.

The write stuff

- Document how long your patient has noted blood in his stool or vomitus and the amount and color of blood (for example, frank red blood, coffee-ground vomitus, or dark-colored or black stool).
- Record the results of your cardiovascular and GI assessments.
- Document your immediate interventions, such as placing the vomiting patient on his side with the head of the bed elevated (if tolerated) and placing the patient on oxygen.
- Frequent vital signs and intake and output may be charted on the frequent vital signs assessment and intake and output sheets.
- Record the name of the practitioner that you notified, the time of notification, orders received, your actions, and the patient's response.
- Document patient teaching and emotional support given.

05/11/06	1315	Upon answering bathroom call light, found pt.
		sitting on toilet, pale, c/o abdominal pain and
		reporting "The toilet is filled with blood."
		Toilet was filled with large amount of bright
		red blood. Assisted pt. to bed. BP 90/50,
		P 114 weak and regular, RR 28, oral T 99° F.
		Pt. placed on O_2 at 2 L/min via NC. Skin
		diaphoretic, cool. Pt. c/o dizziness but alert and
		oriented to time, place, and person. Abdomen
		slightly distended and tender to palpation in
		right upper and lower quadrants. Bowel sounds
		hyperactive. Noted blood seeping from rectum.
		Dr. Cooper notified at 1310 and will be here
		immediately to evaluate pt. —— Deborah Was, RN
05/11/06	1345	Dr. Cooper arrived at 1315 to see pt. and
		new orders written. Lab in to draw blood
		for CBC and electrolytes. I.V. infusion started
		with 20G catheter in Ⓛ antecubital. 1000 ml
		NSS running at 125 ml/hr. Informed consent
		obtained by Dr. Cooper for colonoscopy.
		Reinforced with pt. what to expect before,
		during, and after the procedure. Pt.
		transported to the GI lab at 1345 for
		colonoscopy via stretcher and escorted by
		medical resident. ————— Deborah Was, RN

Health Insurance Portability and Accountability Act

- The Health Insurance Portability and Accountability Act (HIPAA) requires that health care providers, health insurance plans, and government programs (such as Medicare and Medicaid) notify patients about their right to privacy and how their health information will be used and shared.
- Protected health information includes:
  - information in the patient's medical record
  - conversations about the patient's care between health care providers
  - billing information
  - health insurers' computerized records
  - other health information.
- Under HIPAA, the patient has the right to:
  - access his medical information
  - know when health information is shared
  - make changes or corrections to his medical record
  - decide if they want to allow their information to be used for certain purposes, such as marketing or research.
- Patient records with identifiable health information (such as the patient's name, Social Security number, identification

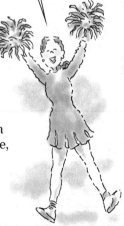

Hip, HIPAA hooray for a patient's right to privacy!

Form fitting

Documenting patient authorization to use personal health information

Your facility probably has an authorization form similar to the one below to be used for release of a patient's personal health information for reasons other than routine treatment or billing. Make sure all the required information is completed before having the patient or legal guardian sign the form.

AUTHORIZATION FORM

By signing, I authorize Community Hospital to use and/or disclose certain protected health information (PHI) about me to ___Dr. Bedarnz___. This authorization permits Community Hospital to use and/or disclose the following individually identifiable health information about me (specifically describe the information to be used or disclosed, such as dates(s) of services, type of services, level of detail to be released, origin of information, etc.):

X-ray films and report, notes on care from 2/6/06 Emergency
Department visit

The information will be used or disclosed for the following purpose:

f/u care with Dr. Bedarnz

(If disclosure is requested by the patient, purpose may be listed as "at the request of the individual.")

The purpose(s) is/are provided so that I can make an informed decision whether to allow release of the information. This authorization will expire on __2/7/06__.
The practice _____ will __X__ will not receive payment or other remuneration from a third party in exchange for using or disclosing the PHI.
I do not have to sign this authorization in order to receive treatment from Community Hospital. In fact, I have the right to refuse to sign this authorization. When my information is used or disclosed pursuant to this authorization, it may be subject to redisclosure by the recipient and may no longer be protected by the federal HIPAA Privacy Rule. I have the right to revoke this authorization in writing except to the extent that the practice has acted in reliance upon this authorization. My written revocation must be submitted to the Privacy Office at:

Community Hospital
123 Main Street
Oakwood, PA

Marcy Thayer	2/6/06	self
Signed by	Date	Relationship to patient
Marcy Thayer		
Print patient's name	Print name of Legal Guardian, if applicable	

number, birth date, admission and discharge dates, and health history) must be secured so that the records aren't accessible to those who don't have a need for them.
- When a patient receives health care, he'll need to sign an authorization form before protected health information can be used for purposes other than routine treatment or billing; this form should be placed in the patient's medical record.
- Use your agency's HIPAA authorization form to document your patient's consent for the use and disclosure of protected health information.

The write stuff
- A HIPAA authorization form must include:
  - description of the health information that will be used and disclosed
  - person authorized to use or disclose the information
  - person to whom the disclosure will be made
  - an expiration date
  - purpose for sharing or using the information
  - signature of the patient or legal guardian.

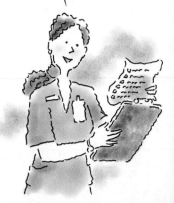

Make sure that the patient has signed the HIPAA authorization form.

Heat application

- Heat applied directly to the patient's body:
  - raises tissue temperature and metabolism
  - enhances the inflammatory process by causing vasodilation and increasing local circulation
  - promotes leukocytosis, suppuration, drainage, and healing
  - reduces pain caused by muscle spasm
  - decreases congestion in deep visceral organs.
- Moist heat softens crusts and exudates.

The write stuff

- Document:
  - date and time of heat application
  - site of application and reason for use
  - type of heat used, such as dry or moist
  - type of device, such as a hot-water bottle, electric heating pad, K pad, chemical hot pack, or warm compresses
  - temperature or heat setting.
- Describe your measures to protect the patient's skin.
- Chart the duration of time the heat was applied.
- Include the condition of the skin before and after the application of heat, and the patient's response to the treatment.
- Record patient teaching provided.

| 11/04/06 | 0900 | Warm moist compress (128° F per bath thermometer) applied to lumbar region of the back for 20 min. for c/o stiffness and discomfort. Skin pink, warm, dry, and intact before application. Told pt. to lay compress over back and not to lie directly on compress. Instructed pt. to call for nurse if he experienced any pain. Skin pink, warm, dry, and intact after the procedure. Pt. reports decrease in stiffness and discomfort. — Brian Petry, RN |

Hyperglycemia

- Defined as an elevated blood glucose level, hyperglycemia results from insufficient insulin or the body's inability to effectively use insulin.
- Extremely high blood glucose levels can lead to ketoacidosis, a potentially life-threatening condition.
- Diabetes mellitus is the most common cause of hyperglycemia, but it may also be attributable to Cushing's syndrome; stresses, such as trauma, infections, burns, and surgery; and drugs such as corticosteroids.
- Patients with diabetes may develop hyperglycemia as a result of insufficient insulin, poor compliance with diet, and illness.
- If your patient develops hyperglycemia, notify the practitioner and anticipate orders for regular insulin therapy and fluid and electrolyte replacement.
- Prompt interventions are necessary to prevent ketoacidosis and a potentially fatal outcome.
- Because caring for a patient with hyperglycemia requires frequent assessments and interventions, document on a timely basis and avoid block charting.

The write stuff

- Record the date and time of your entry.
- Record the patient's blood glucose level.
- Chart your assessment findings, such as polyuria, polydipsia, polyphagia, glycosuria, ketonuria, blurry vision, flushed cheeks, dry skin and mucous membranes, poor skin turgor, weak and rapid pulse, hypotension, Kussmaul's respirations, acetone breath odor, weakness, fatigue, and altered level of consciousness.
- Document the name of the practitioner notified, the time of notification, and the orders received.
- Record your interventions, such as subcutaneous or I.V. administration of regular insulin, frequent blood glucose monitoring, and I.V. fluid and electrolyte replacement.

- Include the patient's response to interventions.
- Use the appropriate flow sheets to record:
  - intake and output
  - I.V. fluids
  - drugs
  - frequent vital signs and blood glucose level.
- Document patient teaching, such as proper nutrition, proper use of insulin, and disease management, provided.

09/29/06	1800	Pt. states, "I vomited and feel weak and dizzy." Face flushed, skin and mucous membranes dry, skin tents when pinched, breath has acetone odor, BP 100/50, P 98 and weak, RR 28 and deep, oral T 98.8° F, blood glucose 462 mg/dl by fingerstick. Dr. Locke notified of findings at 1740 and orders received. I.V. infusion of 1000 ml NSS started in Ⓛ forearm with 22G catheter at 100 ml/hr. Regular insulin 15 units SubQ given in Ⓛ upper arm. Lab called to draw blood for electrolytes and blood glucose levels. Explained rationales for therapy to pt. See flow sheets for frequent documentation of VS, I/O, I.V. fluids, and blood glucose levels. ———————— Ray Barnett, RN
09/29/06	1815	Pt. states, "I'm feeling a little better. I don't feel light-headed any more." BP 118/54, P 94, RR 20, slight acetone odor still noted on breath. Voided 800 ml pale yellow urine, neg. ketones, +2 glucose. ———— Ray Barnett, RN
09/29/06	1830	BP 122/60, P 90 and strong, RR 18. Pt. denies nausea, vomiting, and dizziness. Lab called at 1820 with results of blood draw: blood glucose 375 mg/dl, potassium 3.0 mEq/L. Dr. Locke notified of results at 1825 and order given for 20 mEq of KCL to be added to 1000 ml of NSS to infuse at 100 ml/hr. ———————————— Ray Barnett, RN

Hypertensive crisis

- Hypertensive crisis is a medical emergency in which the patient's diastolic blood pressure suddenly rises above 120 mm Hg.
- Precipitating factors include:
  – abrupt discontinuation of antihypertensive drugs
  – increased salt consumption
  – increased production of renin, epinephrine, and norepinephrine
  – added stress.
- Prompt recognition of hypertensive crisis and nursing interventions to lower blood pressure are vital for preventing stroke, blindness, renal failure, hypertensive encephalopathy, left-sided heart failure, pulmonary edema, and even death.

The write stuff

- Record the date and time of your entry.
- Record the patient's blood pressure.
- Chart the findings of your cardiopulmonary, neurologic, and renal assessments, such as headache, nausea, vomiting, seizures, blurred vision, confusion, drowsiness, heart failure, pulmonary edema, chest pain, and oliguria.
- Document measures to ensure a patent airway.
- Record the:
  – name of the practitioner notified and time of notification
  – orders received, such as continuous blood pressure and cardiac monitoring, I.V. antihypertensive drugs, blood work, supplemental oxygen, and seizure precautions.
- Document the insertion of an arterial line, if applicable.
- Document the patient's response to interventions.
- Use the appropriate flow sheets to record:
  – intake and output
  – drugs
  – frequent vital signs.
- Include patient teaching and emotional support given.

| 03/02/06 | 1200 | Pt. arrived in ED at 1040 with c/o headache, blurred vision, and vomiting. BP 220/120, P 104 bounding, RR 16 unlabored, oral T 97.4° F. Pt. states, "I stopped taking my blood pressure pills 2 days ago when I ran out." Pt. drowsy, but oriented to place and person, knew year but not day of week or time of day. No c/o chest pain, neck veins not distended, lungs clear. Cardiac monitor shows sinus tachycardia, no arrhythmias noted. Dr. Kelly notified and in to see pt. at 1045, orders written. O_2 at 4 L/min. administered via NC. Dr. Kelly explained need for arterial line for BP monitoring. Pt. understands procedure and signed consent. At 1115, assisted Dr. Kelly with insertion of arterial line in Ⓛ radial artery using 20G 2¹/₂″ arterial catheter, after a positive Allen's test. Catheter secured with 1 suture. Transparent semi-permeable dressing applied. Ⓛ hand and wrist secured to arm board. Transducer leveled and zeroed. Initial BP reading 238/124, mean arterial pressure 162 mm Hg with pt.'s head at 30°. Readings accurate to cuff pressures. Line flushes easily. I.V. line inserted in Ⓡ forearm with 18G catheter. Nitroprusside sodium 50 mg in 250 ml D_5W started at 0.3 mcg/kg/min. See frequent vital signs flow sheet for frequent vital signs. Blood sent to lab for stat CBC, ABG, electrolytes, BUN, creatinine, blood glucose level. Stat ECG and portable CXR done, results pending. Foley catheter inserted, urine sent for UA. Side rails padded, bed in low position, airway taped to headboard of bed, suction equipment placed in room. All procedures explained to pt. and wife. Pt. resting comfortably in bed, with HOB at 30°. Pt. states he's no longer nauseated and headache "is much better". ———————— *Paula Walker, RN* |

Hyperthermia-hypothermia blanket

- The hyperthermia-hypothermia blanket is a blanket-sized aquathermia pad that raises, lowers, or maintains body temperature through conductive heat or cold transfer between the blanket and the patient.
- The blanket is used most commonly to reduce high fever when more conservative measures, such as baths, ice packs, and antipyretics, are unsuccessful.
- Other uses include:
  - maintaining normal temperature during surgery or shock
  - inducing hypothermia during surgery to decrease metabolic activity and thereby reduce oxygen requirements
  - reducing intracranial pressure
  - controlling bleeding and intractable pain in patients with amputations, burns, or cancer
  - providing warmth in cases of severe hypothermia.

The write stuff

- Record the date and time of your entry.
- Document that the procedure was explained to the patient.
- Document that a consent form was signed, if required by your facility.
- Record:
  - vital signs
  - neurologic signs
  - fluid intake and output
  - skin condition
  - position change.
- Using the appropriate flow sheets and per your facility's policy, record vital signs and the findings of your neurologic assessment:
  - every 5 minutes until the desired body temperature is reached
  - and then every 15 minutes until the temperature is stable or as ordered.

- Document:
  - type of hyperthermia-hypothermia unit (manual or automatic) used
  - control and temperature settings.
- Note the duration of the procedure and the patient's tolerance of treatment.
- Describe measures taken to prevent skin injury.
- Record signs of complications such as shivering, marked changes in vital signs, increased intracranial pressure, respiratory distress or arrest, cardiac arrest, oliguria, anuria.
- Record:
  - name of the practitioner notified of complications
  - time of notification
  - orders received
  - your actions
  - patient's response.

01/19/06	1000	Need for hypothermia blanket explained to pt.'s wife by Dr. Albright. Wife signed consent form. Preprocedure VS: Rectal T 104.3° F, P 112 and regular, RR 28, BP 138/88. Automatic hypothermia blanket, set at 99° F, placed under pt. at 0945. Sheet placed between pt. and hypothermia blanket. Lanolin applied to back, buttocks, and undersides of legs, arms, and feet. Skin intact, flushed, warm to the touch. Rectal probe in place and secured with tape. Pt. drowsy, but easily arousable and oriented to place and person but not time, able to feel light touch in all extremities, moving all extremities on own, no c/o numbness or tingling, PEARLA. See I/O and frequent vital signs flow sheets for hourly intake and output, and q5min. VS and neuro. assessments. No shivering noted, Foley catheter intact draining clear amber urine, no dyspnea. ———————————————— Jane Waters, RN

Hypoglycemia

- Occurring when the blood glucose level drops below 60 mg/dl, hypoglycemia is a potentially fatal metabolic disorder.
- Hypoglycemia may occur as a complication of diabetes mellitus, but also as a result of adrenal insufficiency, myxedema, poor nutrition, hepatic disease, alcoholism, vigorous exercise, and certain drugs such as pentamidine.
- If your patient is hypoglycemic, obtain a blood glucose level, immediately notify the practitioner, and administer a carbohydrate or glucagon, as ordered, to prevent irreversible brain damage and death.

The write stuff

- Record the date and time of your entry.
- Record your patient's signs and symptoms of hypoglycemia, such as hunger, weakness, shakiness, paresthesia, nervousness, palpitations, tachycardia, diaphoresis, and pallor, or with more severe hypoglycemia, drowsiness, reduced level of consciousness, slurred speech, behavior changes, incoordination, seizures, and coma.
- Document the results of the blood glucose level determined by fingerstick.
- Note the name of the practitioner notified, the time of notification, and the orders received.
- Record:
    – route (oral, I.V., or subcutaneous) of carbohydrate given
    – type and amount of carbohydrate given
    – patient's response.
- If repeat doses are necessary, write a separate note for each administration, including the patient's response.
- Record all repeat blood glucose determinations and the measurement method used.
- Document other interventions, such as maintaining a patent airway and seizure precautions, and the patient's response.

- Use the appropriate flow sheets to record:
  - intake and output
  - I.V. fluids
  - drugs
  - frequent vital signs and blood glucose levels.
- Document patient teaching provided, such as signs and symptoms of hypoglycemia, treating hypoglycemic episodes, preventive measures to avoid hypoglycemia, and disease management.

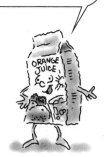

Keep track of those carbs! Chart the route used, type given, and the patient's response.

07/19/06	1850	While performing p.m. care at 1840, noted pt. had slurred speech and shaky hands. When questioned, pt. stated, "I feel okay. I just have a little headache." Pt. stated she wasn't very hungry at dinner. P 108, RR 14, BP 110/60, oral T 97.4° F. Skin pale and diaphoretic. Denies paresthesia. Received glyburide 5 mg at 1700. Blood glucose level by fingerstick 62 mg/dl. Dr. Luu notified at 1845 and ordered 15 g of oral carbohydrate. Gave 1/2 cup of orange juice. ———— Ani Franco, RN
07/19/06	1900	Blood glucose level 71 mg/dl by fingerstick. Speech remains slurred, skin pale and diaphoretic, denies paresthesia, still c/o headache. P 104, RR16, BP 118/70. Gave pt. an additional 1/2 cup orange juice. ———— Ani Franco, RN
07/19/06	1915	Blood glucose level by fingerstick 98 mg/dl. P 88, RR 16, BP 118/68. Speech clear, skin pink, slight diaphoresis noted, reports headache gone. Pt. states, "I feel much better. I didn't know my blood sugar was so low." Explained relationship between oral hypoglycemic and timing of meals, reviewed s/s of hypoglycemia and its treatment. ———— Ani Franco, RN

Hypotension

- Defined as blood pressure below 90/60 mm Hg, hypotension reduces perfusion to the tissues and organs of the body.
- Severe hypotension is a medical emergency that may progress to shock and death.
- Hypotension may be caused by:
  - various disorders of the cardiopulmonary, neurologic, and metabolic systems
  - use of certain drugs
  - stress
  - position changes
  - changes in heart rhythm, the pumping action of the heart, and fluid balance.
- Because hypotension can be fatal, prompt recognition and interventions are necessary.
  - Notify the practitioner immediately, insert an I.V. line to administer fluids, begin cardiac monitoring, and administer oxygen.
  - Anticipate administering vasopressor drugs and hemodynamic monitoring.

The write stuff

- Record the date and time of your entry.
- Record your patient's blood pressure and other vital signs.
- Document your assessment findings, such as bradycardia, tachycardia, weak pulses, oliguria, reduced bowel sounds, dizziness, syncope, reduced level of consciousness, myocardial ischemia, and cool, clammy skin.
- Note the name of the practitioner notified, the time of notification, and orders received, such as continuous blood pressure and cardiac monitoring, obtaining a 12-lead electrocardiogram, administering supplemental oxygen, and inserting an I.V. line for fluids and vasopressor drugs.

- Describe other interventions, such as lowering the head of the bed, inserting an indwelling urinary catheter, and assisting with insertion of hemodynamic monitoring lines.
- Document adherence to advanced cardiac life support (ACLS) protocols (if hypotension is caused by an arrhythmia), using a code sheet to record interventions, if necessary.
- Use the appropriate flow sheets to record:
  – intake and output
  – I.V. fluids
  – drugs
  – frequent vital signs.
- Record the patient's responses to interventions.
- Include emotional support and patient teaching provided.

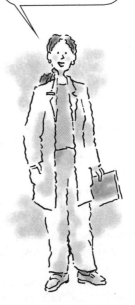

With hypotension, you may need to use a code sheet to document that you followed ACLS protocols.

| 08/01/06 | 1235 | Pt. c/o dizziness at 1220. P 48, RR 18, BP 86/48, oral T 97.6° F. Peripheral pulses weak, skin cool and diaphoretic, normal bowel sounds, clear breath sounds, alert and oriented to time, place, and person, no c/o chest pain. Continuous cardiac monitoring via portable monitor shows failure of permanent pacemaker to capture. Rhythm strip mounted below. Dr. Luther called at 1225, came to see pt., and orders received. 12-lead ECG done and confirms failure to capture. Pt. placed on O₂ 2 L by NC. Intermittent infusion device started in ® forearm with 18G catheter. VS recorded q5min on frequent VS sheet. Stat portable CXR done at 1230. Explained pacemaker malfunction to pt. Assured her that she's being monitored and that a temporary pacemaker is available, if needed. Dr. Luther called pt.'s husband and told him of situation. ———— *Martha Kent, RN* |

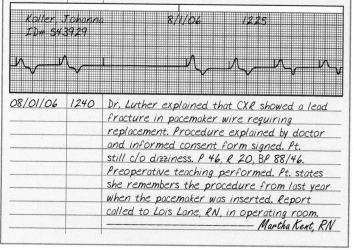

Koller, Johanna
ID# 543929
8/1/06   1225

| 08/01/06 | 1240 | Dr. Luther explained that CXR showed a lead fracture in pacemaker wire requiring replacement. Procedure explained by doctor and informed consent form signed. Pt. still c/o dizziness. P 46, R 20, BP 88/46. Preoperative teaching performed. Pt. states she remembers the procedure from last year when the pacemaker was inserted. Report called to Lois Lane, RN, in operating room. ———— *Martha Kent, RN* |

Hypovolemia

- When a patient is hypovolemic, reduced intravascular blood volume causes circulatory dysfunction and inadequate tissue perfusion.
- Without sufficient blood or fluid replacement, the patient develops hypovolemic shock, which can progress to irreversible cerebral and renal damage, cardiac arrest and, ultimately, death.
- The most common cause of hypovolemic shock is acute blood loss.
- Other causes include severe burns, intestinal obstruction, peritonitis, acute pancreatitis, ascites, dehydration from excessive perspiration, severe diarrhea or protracted vomiting, diabetes insipidus, diuresis, and inadequate fluid intake.
- If your patient is hypovolemic, assess for and maintain a patent airway, breathing, and circulation.
- Expect to administer blood or fluid replacement and well as inotropic and vasopressor drugs.
- Other nursing interventions focus on identifying and treating the underlying cause.

The write stuff

- Record the date and time of your entry.
- Record your assessment findings, such as hypotension; tachycardia; rapid, shallow respirations; reduced urine output; cold, pale, clammy skin; weight loss; poor skin turgor; weak, diminished, or absent pulses; and reduced level of consciousness.
- Record the name of the practitioner notified, the time of notification, and orders received.

- Document interventions to ensure a patent airway, breathing, and circulation, and the patient's responses.
- Chart your actions, such as:
  - continuous blood pressure and cardiac monitoring
  - I.V. inotropic and vasopressor drugs
  - I.V. blood and fluid replacement
  - blood work
  - supplemental oxygen
  - assisting with insertion of hemodynamic monitoring lines.
- Chart the patient's response to interventions.
- Use the appropriate flow sheets to record:
  - intake and output
  - I.V. fluids
  - drugs
  - frequent vital signs.
- Include patient teaching and emotional support given.

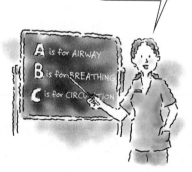

When documenting hypovolemia, include what you did to ensure the ABCs.

A is for AIRWAY
B is for BREATHING
C is for CIRCULATION

10/17/06	1415	Pt. restless and confused to time and place. P 120 reg, BP 88/58, RR 28 shallow, rectal T 96.8° F. Lungs clear, neck veins flat, skin cold and clammy and tents when pinched, peripheral pulses weak. Urine output last hour 25 ml via Foley catheter. Placed pt. flat in bed on Ⓛ side. Pt. placed on O₂ at 4 L via NC. Notified Dr. Parker of findings at 1410, came to see pt., and orders written. Continuous cardiac monitoring shows sinus tachycardia. Automated cuff placed for continuous BP monitoring. ———————————— Andrew Williams, RN
10/17/06	1450	Dr. Parker explained need for hemodynamic monitoring to pt.'s husband, who signed consent. Assisted Dr. Parker with insertion of pulmonary artery catheter into Ⓡ subclavian vein at 1430. Pressures on insertion: CVP 2 mm Hg, PAD 4 mm Hg, PAWP 3 mm Hg. Wedge tracing obtained with 1.5 ml balloon inflation. NSS 1000 ml at 120 ml/hr infusing in proximal infusion port. Using flush solution of 500 units heparin in 500 ml NSS. Catheter sutured in place and site covered with transparent semipermeable dressing. Portable CXR confirmed line placement. Lab in to draw blood for CBC, electrolytes, BUN, creatinine, serum lactate, and coagulation studies at 1445. ———————————— Andrew Williams, RN
10/17/06	1500	ABG drawn by Thomas Reilly, RPT, at 1450. O₂ at 4 L via NC w/ pulse oximetry of 95%. See flow sheets for frequent VS, I/O, and hemodynamic readings. All procedures explained to pt. and husband. Pt. lying comfortably in bed, oriented to time, place, and person. Given Tylenol 650 mg p.o. at 1455 for mild discomfort at catheter insertion site. ———— ———————————— Andrew Williams, RN

Hypoxemia

- Defined as a low concentration of oxygen in the arterial blood, hypoxemia occurs when the partial pressure of arterial oxygen (PaO_2) falls below 60 mm Hg.
- Hypoxemia causes poor tissue perfusion and may lead to respiratory failure.
- Hypoxemia may be caused by a condition that results in:
  - hypoventilation abnormalities (such as head trauma, stroke, or central nervous system depressant drugs)
  - diffusion abnormalities (including pulmonary edema, pulmonary fibrosis, and emphysema)
  - ventilation/perfusion mismatches (such as chronic obstructive pulmonary disease or restrictive lung disorders)
  - shunting of blood (such as pneumonia, atelectasis, acute respiratory distress syndrome, pulmonary edema, and pulmonary embolism).
- If you suspect your patient is hypoxemic, notify the practitioner immediately and anticipate interventions to prevent and treat respiratory failure.

The write stuff

- Record the date and time of your entry.
- Record your patient's PaO_2 level.
- Document cardiopulmonary assessment findings, such as change in level of consciousness, tachycardia, increased blood pressure, tachypnea, dyspnea, mottled skin, cyanosis, and, in patients with severe hypoxemia, bradycardia and hypotension.
- Chart the name of the practitioner notified, the time of notification, and orders received.
- Record your interventions, such as:
  - measuring oxygen saturation by pulse oximetry
  - obtaining arterial blood gas values

- providing supplemental oxygen
- positioning the patient in a high Fowler's position
- assisting with endotracheal intubation
- monitoring mechanical ventilation
- providing continuous cardiac monitoring.
- Document the patient's responses to interventions.
- Use the appropriate flow sheets to record:
  - intake and output
  - I.V. fluids
  - drugs
  - frequent vital signs.
- Include emotional support and patient teaching provided.

| 07/19/06 | 1400 | At 1330, pt. found restless and confused, SOB, skin mottled. P 112, BP 148/78, RR 32 labored, rectal T 97.4° F. Dr. Moreau notified of findings at 1335 and came to see pt. at 1345. ABGs drawn by doctor and sent to lab. Pulse oximetry 86% on O2 3 L/min by NC. Placed on O$_2$ 100% via nonrebreather mask with pulse oximetry 92%. Pt. positioned in high Fowler's position. Continuous cardiac monitoring shows sinus tachycardia at 116, no arrhythmias noted. Radiology called for stat portable CXR. Dr. Moreau notified wife of change in husband's status. See VS and IO flowsheets for frequent assessments. ————— Kim D'Amico, RN |

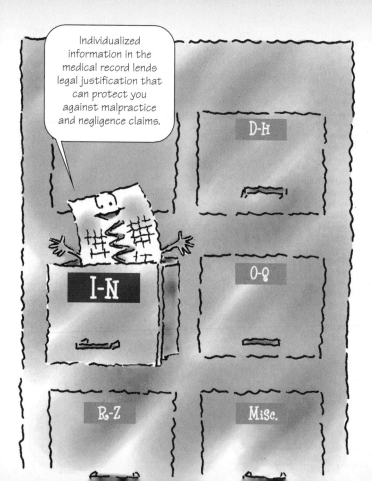

IJK

Illegal drug possession

- If you observe that your patient has illegal drugs or drug paraphernalia in his possession:
  - follow your facility's policy
  - notify your nursing supervisor, security, and the patient's practitioner.
- Depending on your state's guidelines, you may be obligated to report the patient to the police.

Making a case

Conducting a drug search

If you suspect your patient is abusing drugs or you discover drugs in the patient's possession, you have a duty to do something about it. If the patient harms himself or anyone else, resulting in a lawsuit, the court may hold you liable for his actions.

Known drug abuse
- You may find drugs in a patient's possession (for example, in the emergency department while looking for identification in the patient's clothes or handbag).
- In this situation, facility policy may obligate you to:
  - confiscate the drugs

  - take steps to ensure that the patient doesn't acquire more.

Suspected drug abuse
- If a patient's erratic or threatening behavior makes you suspect drug abuse, consult your facility's policy and notify your nursing supervisor, who may direct you to conduct a search.
- You may be safe legally to perform the search if you:
  - strongly believe the patient poses a threat to himself or others
  - can document your reasons for searching his possessions.

Conducting a drug search *(continued)*

Guidelines for searches
• Before you conduct a search, review your facility's guidelines.
• Most facility guidelines first direct you to contact your supervisor and explain why you have legitimate cause for a search.
• If you receive approval for the search, ask a security guard to help you. Besides protecting you, he'll serve as a witness if you do find drugs.
• When you're ready, confront the patient, tell him you intend to conduct a search, and tell him why.
• Depending on your facility's guidelines, you can search a patient's belongings as well as his room.

• If you find illegal drugs during your search, confiscate them. In addition, your facility policy may obligate you to take steps to ensure that the patient doesn't acquire more.
• Possession of illegal drugs is a felony. Depending on your facility's guidelines, you may be obligated to report the patient to the police.

Documenting the search
• Record your findings in your nurse's note and in an incident report.
• Your written records will be an important part of your defense (and your facility's) if the patient decides to sue.

The write stuff
• Record the date and time of your entry.
• If you discover evidence of drugs in your patient's room or on his person, document the circumstances of the discovery.
• Document that you told the patient about the facility's policy on contraband; include the patient's response.
• Record:
  – names and departments of the people you notified
  – instructions received
  – your actions.
• Document:
  – whether a search was performed
  – who performed it

- who was present during the search
- what was found (for example, pills, liquid, or powder as
  well as the amount, color, and shape).
- Fill out a form to report the occurrence, according to your
  facility's policy.

09/01/06	1000	Clear plastic bag containing white powdery
		substance, approx. 3 tbsp, with odd odor
		found in pt.'s bedside stand while retrieving
		his wash basin at 0930. Upon questioning, pt.
		stated, "That stuff is none of your business."
		Told pt. that drugs not prescribed by the
		doctor aren't allowed in the hospital. Security
		director, Michael Daniels; nursing supervisor,
		Stacey McLean, RN; and Dr. Phillips notified at
		0940. Mr. Daniels and Mrs. McLean visited pt.
		in his room and reinforced hospital policy on
		contraband. Pt. flushed powder down toilet.
		Witnessed by Mr. Daniels, Mrs. McLean, and
		myself. Dr. Phillips will see pt. at 1030 to
		discuss situation. ———————— Greg Little, RN

Incident report

- An incident is an event that's inconsistent with the facility's ordinary routine, regardless of whether injury occurs.
- In most health care facilities, incident reports are required for:
  - any injury to a patient, employee, or visitor
  - patient complaints
  - medication errors.
- An incident report:
  - informs hospital administration of the incident so that it can monitor patterns and trends, thereby helping to prevent future similar incidents (risk management).
  - alerts administration and the hospital's insurance company to the possibility of liability claims and the need for further investigation (claims management).
- Complete an incident report immediately after the incident to ensure accurate reporting of details.
- Don't document in the patient's medical record that an incident report was filed.

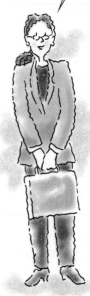

Incident reports play a role in risk management and claims management.

The write stuff

- When filing an incident report, include only:
  - the date and exact time and place of the incident
  - the names of the persons involved and any witnesses
  - factual information about what happened and the known consequences to the person involved
  - any relevant facts, such as your immediate actions in response to the incident (for example, notifying the patient's practitioner).

Help desk

Tips for writing an incident report

Write objectively
Record the details of the incident in objective terms, describing exactly what you saw and heard. For example, unless you actually saw a patient fall, write: "Found patient lying on the floor." Then describe only the actions you took to provide care at the scene, such as helping the patient back into bed, assessing him for injuries, and calling the practitioner.

Avoid opinions
Don't commit your opinions to writing in the incident report.

Assign no blame
Don't admit to liability and don't blame or point your finger at colleagues or administrators. Steer clear of such statements as "Better staffing would have prevented this incident." State only what happened.

Avoid hearsay and assumptions
Include the names of the people involved, any witnesses to the event, and their factual statements about the incident.

File the report properly
Don't file the incident report with the patient's medical record. Send the report to the person designated to review it according to your facility's policy.

- Sign and date the report.
- Write a factual account of the incident in the patient's medical record, including the treatment, follow-up care, and the patient's response.
- Include in the progress note and in the incident report anything the patient or his family says about their role in the incident.

Form fitting

Completing an incident report

When you discover a reportable event, you must fill out an incident report. Forms vary but most include the following information.

INCIDENT REPORT

Date of incident _6-25-06_

Time of incident _1300_

Name _Erin Fanning_
Address _7 Worth Way, Bensalem, PA_
Phone _(215) 555-1122_

Exact location of incident (Bldg, Floor, Room No, Area) _3B-Room 310_

Type of incident (check only one)
☑Patient ☐Employee ☐Visitor ☐Volunteer ☐Other (specify) _____

Description of incident (who, what, when, where, how, why)
(Use back of form if necessary) _Pt. found on floor next to bed. Pt._
stated, "I was trying to reach my slippers and lost my balance."

Patient fall incidents	Floor conditions: ☑Clean and smooth ☐Slippery (wet) ☐Other: _____
	Frame of bed: ☑Low ☐High │ Other restraints (type and extent): _N/A_
	Were bed rails present?: ☐No ☑1 up ☐2 up ☐3 up ☐4 up │ Night light?: ☐Yes ☑No
	Ambulation privilege: ☑Unlimited ☐Limited with assistance ☐Complete bedrest ☐Other: _____
	Were opioids, analgesics, hypnotics, sedatives, diuretics, antihypertensives, or anticonvulsants given during last 4 hours? ☐Yes ☑No Drug: _____ Amount: _____ Time: _____
Patient incidents	Physician notified (Complete if applicable): Name of physician: _C. Chaplin, MD_ Date: _06/25/06_ Time: _1310_

(continued)

Completing an incident report *(continued)*

Employee incidents	Department _____ Job title _____ Social security # _____ Marital status _____	

All incidents	Notified: _L. Savage, RN_ Date: _6/25/06_ Time: _1310_ Location where treatment was rendered: _____

Name, address and telephone numbers of witness(es) or persons familiar with incident — witness or not:

Janet Petkov, (215) 555-0912, 1 Main St., Bensalem, PA

_____

Signature of person preparing report: _Leah Savage_ Title: _RN_
Date of report: _6/25/06_

Physician's report — To be completed for all cases involving injury or illness (do not use abbreviations) (Use back if necessary)
Diagnosis and treatment: _____

_____

_____

Disposition: _____

Person notified other than hospital personnel: _____

Date: _____ Time: _____

Name and address: _____

Physician's signature: _____ Date:_____

Infection control

- Various federal agencies require documentation of infections so that the data can be assessed and used to help prevent and control future infections.
- The data you record helps your health care facility meet national and local accreditation standards.
- Typically, you must report to your facility's infection control department any:
  - culture result that shows a positive infection
  - surgery, drug, fever, X-ray finding, or specific treatment related to infection.

The write stuff

- Record the date and time of your entry.
- Record that you followed standard precautions against direct contact with blood and body fluids.
- If indicated, document that you followed transmission-based precautions, such as airborne, droplet, and contact precautions.
- Record the dates and times of your interventions in the patient's chart and on the Kardex.
- Document any breach in an isolation technique, and file an incident report should such a breach occur.
- Note the:
  - name of the doctor and infection control practitioner that you notified of the results of any suspected infection or culture and sensitivity results
  - time of notification
  - orders received, such as administration of drugs to treat the infection.
- Record the patient's response to interventions.

- Record patient education provided, such as:
  - steps for maintaining standard precautions
  - steps for maintaining transmission-based precautions, if indicated
  - signs and symptoms of infection to report
  - importance of taking drugs as prescribed.

11/21/06	1300	Standard and contact precautions maintained. P 96, BP 132/82, rectal T 102.3° F. Large amount of purulent yellow-green, foul-smelling drainage from incision soaked through 6 4" X 4" gauze pads in 2 hr. Dr. Spohn notified at 1250. Ordered Tylenol 650 mg P.O. q 4 hr prn for temp greater than 101.7° F; given at 1250. Repeat C&S obtained and sent to lab. Wound cleaned w/NSS and covered with 4 sterile 4" X 4" pads using sterile technique. Reinforced standard and contact precautions to pt. and wife. Jill Hayden, infection control RN notified of infection at 1255 and will be here w/in the hour to review the medical record. ———————— Linda Sobolewski, RN

Informed consent, inability to provide

- Informed consent relies on an individual's capacity or ability to make decisions at a particular time under specific circumstances.
- A person must possess the capacity and the competence to make medical decisions.
- If you have reason to believe that a patient isn't competent to participate in giving consent because of a medical condition or sedation, you have an obligation to bring it to the practitioner's attention immediately.
- If the practitioner has discussed consent issues with the patient at a time when the patient was heavily sedated or medicated, you need to bring your concerns to the practitioner's attention or to your supervisor's attention if the practitioner isn't available.

Making a case

When a patient can't give proper consent

If you believe your patient isn't competent to participate in giving consent because of medication or sedation and you do nothing, and the patient undergoes the procedure without giving proper consent, you might find yourself as a co-defendant in a battery lawsuit. The patient may sue for lack of informed consent due to temporary lack of capacity.

Record review

Patient's lawyers, judges, and juries will look closely at the medication records to see when, in relation to the signing of the consent form, the patient was last medicated and the patient's response to the medication. You could be held jointly responsible for the patient undergoing a procedure that he didn't consent to if:

- you took part in the battery by assisting with the treatment
- you knew it was taking place and you didn't try to stop it.

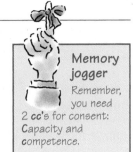

- If the patient can't provide consent, follow facility policy on contacting legal guardians or family members for consent before the procedure is performed.

The write stuff

- Record the date and time of your note.
- Document conversations with the patient, including his:
  - mental status
  - understanding of the procedure, complications, and expected outcomes.
- Record whether:
  - your patient is confused or medicated
  - you can't provide the information the patient needs
  - the patient doesn't understand the procedure
  - you assessed that the patient wasn't competent to provide consent when speaking with the practitioner because of medication or sedation.
- Record the names of the practitioner and nursing supervisor that you notified, the times of notification, and their responses.

| 07/19/06 | 0700 | Pt. given morphine 4 mg I.V. push at 0630 for chest pain. Dr. Turk in to see pt. at 0645 to explain cardiac cath procedure and obtain informed consent. Pt. keeps asking, "Where am I? What is happening?" Dr. Turk explained that she was in CCU with chest pain and was scheduled for a cardiac catheterization this a.m. Pt. keeps asking, "What is this test and why do I need it?" Dr. Turk cancelled cardiac cath. for this a.m. Doctor will come back to see pt. later today. ———————— Tracy Diehl, R.N. |

Informed consent in an emergency

- A patient must sign a consent form before most treatments and procedures.
- Informed consent means that the patient understands the proposed therapy, alternative therapies, the risks, and the hazards of not undergoing any treatment at all.
- Emergency treatment may be done without first obtaining consent in specific circumstances:
  - to save a patient's life
  - to prevent loss of organ, limb, or a function
  - if the patient is unconscious
  - if the patient is a minor who can't give consent.
- The presumption in an emergency is that the patient would have consented if he had been able.
- For example, to sustain the life of unconscious patients in the emergency department, intubation has been held to be appropriate even if no one is available to consent to the procedure.
- Courts will uphold emergency medical treatment as long as:
  - reasonable effort was made to obtain consent
  - no alternative treatments were available to save life or limb.

The write stuff

- Record the date and time of your entry.
- Document the emergency and the reason your patient can't give informed consent (such as being unconscious).
- Describe efforts to reach family members to obtain consent.
- List the names, addresses, telephone numbers, and relationships of the people you or the practitioner attempted to reach.
- Record that no alternative treatment was available to save life or limb.

08/19/06	1000	Pt. arrived in ED at 0940 via ambulance
		following MVC. Pt. not responding to verbal
		commands, opens eyes and pushes at stimulus
		in response to pain, making no verbal
		responses. Pt. has bruising across upper chest,
		labored breathing, skin pale and cool, normal S_1
		and S_2 heart sounds, diminished breath sounds
		throughout ® lung, normal breath sounds Ⓛ
		lung, no tracheal deviation. P 112, BP 88/52, RR
		26. Dr. Keaton called at 0945 and came to see
		pt. I.V. line inserted in Ⓛ antecubital with
		20G catheter. 1000 ml NSS infusing at 125
		ml/hr. 100% oxygen given via nonrebreather
		mask. Stat CXR ordered to confirm
		pneumothorax. Pt. identified by driver's license
		and credit cards as Michael Brown of 123
		Maple St., Valley View. Dr. Keaton called house
		to speak with family about need for immediate
		chest tube and treatment, no answer, left
		message on machine. Business card of Michelle
		Brown found in wallet. Company receptionist
		confirms she is wife of Michael Brown, but
		she's out of the office and won't return until
		this afternoon. Left message at 0945 for wife
		to call doctor. ———————— Heidi Lipa, RN
08/19/06	1015	At 0955 noted tracheal deviation to Ⓛ side,
		difficulty breathing, cyanosis of lips, and
		mucous membranes, distended neck veins,
		absent breath sounds in ® lung, muffled heart
		sounds. P 120, BP 88/58, RR 32. Pt.'s
		neurologic status unchanged. Dr. Keaton
		ordered chest tube to be inserted on ® side
		to relieve tension pneumothorax. Because of
		pt.'s deteriorating condition, pt. was unable to
		give consent. At 1010, Dr. Keaton called pt.'s
		home and wife's place of business but was
		unable to speak with her. Dr. Keaton left
		messages to return his call. ——— Heidi Lipa, RN

Informed consent for a minor

- Informed consent involves ensuring that the patient or someone acting on his behalf has enough information to know the risks and benefits of a treatment, procedure, drug, or surgery.
- When the patient is a minor, the practitioner must give a full explanation of care to the parent or designated adult responsible for signing the consent.
- Ethically, nurses have a duty to inform a minor of the procedure and risks and involve him in decisions regardless of whether he can consent to care.
- When controversies arise and a court hearing ensues, the older the minor is, the more likely his wishes will be followed.

The write stuff

- Record the date and time consent was given.
- Describe the involvement of the child and other persons present.
- Record any questions or comments that the child, parents, or significant others had.
- Ask the responsible adult and the child to restate the purpose of the procedure, drug, or surgery in their own words and record their responses.
- Describe any teaching done with the adults and child.

| 11/12/06 | 1420 | Consent obtained by Dr. Dautrieve for Bobby Hill's tonsillectomy from Mr. and Mrs. Hill, parents of Bobby, at 1400 at the preop clinic appt. Parents were able to state the purpose of the surgery and the risks involved. Asked Bobby to draw a picture of his surgery and he drew a picture of the operating room with the doctor "pulling out" his tonsils. When asked how he felt about having the surgery, he said, "I'll be glad to go to swim practice again." ———— ———————————————————— Christina Yang, R.N |

Intake and output

- Many patients, including surgical patients, those on I.V. therapy, and those with fluid and electrolyte imbalances, burns, hemorrhage, or edema, require 24-hour intake and output monitoring.
- This information is typically documented on an intake and output record.
- For easy reference, list the volumes of standard containers, such as styrofoam cups or milk containers.
- Delivery devices make documenting enteral and I.V. intake more accurate.
- You must make sure that the patient, family members, and other caregivers understand how to record or report all foods and fluids that the patient consumes orally, even if the patient receives them in other departments.
- Include I.V. piggyback infusions, drugs given by I.V. push, patient-controlled analgesics, and any irrigation solutions that aren't withdrawn.
- If the patient is ambulatory, remind him to use a urinal or a commode.
- The normal amount of fluid lost through the GI tract (100 ml or less daily) isn't accounted for on the intake and output form; however, if the patient's stools become excessive or watery, they must be counted as output.

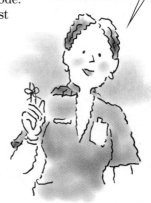

Don't forget to count lost fluids such as vomit, drainage, and blood on intake and output records.

Form fitting

Intake and output record

As the sample shows, you can monitor your patient's fluid balance by using an intake and output record.

Patient's name: _Meredith Grey_
Medical record #: _49731_
Admission date: _2/14/06_

INTAKE AND OUTPUT RECORD

Date: 02/15/06	Intake					
	Oral	Tube feeding	Instilled	I.V. and IVPB	TPN	**Total**
0700–1500	250	320	H_2O 50	1100		1720
1500–2300	200	320	H_2O 50	1100		1670
2300–0700		320	H_2O 50	1100		1470
24 hr total	450	960	H_2O 150	3300		4860

Date: 02/15/06	Output				
	Urine	Emesis tube	NG tube	Other	**Total**
0700–1500	1355		100		1455
1500–2300	1200		50		1250
2300–0700	1500		100		1600
24 hr total	4055		250		4305

Standard measures:
Styrofoam cup . . . . 240 ml
Juice . . . . 120 ml
Milk (small) . . . . 120 ml
Water (small) . . . . 120 ml
Water (large) . . . . 600 ml
Water pitcher . . . . 750 ml
Coffee . . . . 240 ml
Soup . . . . 180 ml
Ice cream or gelatin . . 120 ml

Key:
IVPB = I.V. piggyback
TPN = total parenteral nutrition
NG = nasogastric

- Other measurable sources of fluid loss include:
  – vomiting
  – drainage from suction devices and wound drains
  – bleeding.
- If the patient is incontinent, document this as well as tube drainage and irrigation volumes.

The write stuff

- Write your patient's name on the intake and output record.
- Record the date and time of your shift on the appropriate line.
- Record the total intake and output for each category of fluid for your shift, then total these categories and provide a shift total for intake and output.
  – At the end of 24 hours, a daily total is calculated, usually by the night nurse, and recorded on the intake and output record.
- Use a consistent unit of measurement, in most cases, milliliters.
- Document any patient education provided in your narrative note.

Intestinal obstruction

- An intestinal obstruction is a partial or complete blockage of the lumen in the small or large bowel.
- Intestinal obstructions are most likely to occur from adhesions caused by previous abdominal surgery, external hernias, volvulus, Crohn's disease, radiation enteritis, intestinal wall hematomas, and neoplasms.
- When your patient has an intestinal obstruction, assess and treat him for peritonitis and shock, life-threatening conditions.
- Anticipate administering I.V. fluids, electrolytes, blood, and antibiotics.
- Assist with insertion of a nasogastric or intestinal tube for decompression of the bowel.
- Prepare your patient for surgery, if necessary.

The write stuff

- Record the date and time of your entry.
- Record the results of your GI assessment, such as colicky pain, abdominal tenderness, rebound tenderness, nausea, vomiting, constipation, liquid stools, borborygmi or absent bowel sounds, and abdominal distention.
- Chart the results of your cardiopulmonary, renal, and neurologic assessments.
- Document:
  - name of the practitioner notified and time of notification
  - orders received
  - your actions and the patient's response to them.
- Use the appropriate flow sheets to record:
  - intake and output
  - I.V. fluids and drugs administered
  - frequent vital signs.
- Record:
  - type of decompression tube inserted
  - name of the practitioner inserting the tube
  - suction type and amount

- color, amount, and consistency of drainage
- mouth and nose care provided
- patient's tolerance of the procedure.
- Document:
  - patient's level of pain on a scale of 0 to 10, with 10 being the worst pain imaginable
  - your interventions and the patient's response to them.
- Record all drugs given on the medication administration record and document the patient's response to them in your note.
- Document patient education and emotional support given.

09/19/06	1810	Pt. c/o nausea and cramping abdominal pain.
		Vomited 150 ml green liquid. States he hasn't
		had BM X 5 days. P 112, BP 128/72, RR 28, oral
		T 99.0° F. Abdominal exam shows rebound
		tenderness, distention, and high-pitched
		hyperactive bowel sounds. Pt. is alert and
		oriented to time, place, and person. Normal
		heart sounds. Breath sounds clear. Skin pale,
		cool, peripheral pulses palpable. Voiding
		approx. 400 ml q4hr. Notified Dr. Webber at
		1745 of these findings. Orders given. Pt. NPO.
		Explained NPO to pt. and wife, answered their
		questions, and explained treatments being
		done. Stat abdominal X-ray done at 1755. Lab
		in to draw blood for electrolytes, BUN,
		creatinine, CBC w/diff. at 1800. I.V. infusion
		started in Ⓡ forearm with 18G catheter. 1000
		ml of D5NSS w/KCL 20 mEq/L infusing at
		75 ml/hr. Dr. Webber in at 1805 to explain
		possible bowel obstruction to pt. and wife.
		Dr. Webber told them that depending on the
		results of X-ray, pt. may need decompression
		tube, and explained to them the reasons for
		this treatment. See I.V., I/O, and VS flow
		sheets. ——————— Isabel Stevens, RN

I.V. catheter insertion

- Peripheral I.V. line insertion involves selecting a venipuncture device and an insertion site, preparing the site, and inserting a device.
- Selection of a venipuncture device and site depends on:
  - type of solution to be used
  - frequency and duration of infusion
  - patency and location of accessible veins
  - patient's age, size, and condition
  - when possible, the patient's preference.
- I.V. catheters are inserted to administer medications, blood, or blood products or to correct fluid and electrolyte imbalances.

The write stuff

- In your note or on the appropriate I.V. sheets, record the date and time of the venipuncture.
- Include the type, gauge, and length of the needle or catheter as well as the anatomic location of the insertion site.
- Document the number of attempts at venipuncture (if you made more than one).
- Indicate the type and flow rate of the I.V. solution, the name and amount of medication in the solution (if any), and any adverse reactions and actions taken to correct them.

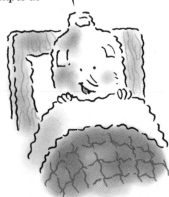

Check out my I.V. sheets!

- If the I.V. site was changed, document the reason for the change.
- Document patient teaching given and evidence of patient understanding.

10/03/06	1100	20G 1½" catheter inserted in Ⓡ forearm
		without difficulty on the first attempt. Site
		dressed with transparent dressing and tape.
		I.V. infusion of 1000 ml D5W started at
		100 ml/hr. I.V. infusing without difficulty.
		Pt. instructed to notify nurse if the site
		becomes swollen or painful, or catheter
		becomes dislodged or leaks. No c/o pain
		after insertion. ——— Preston Burke, R.N

I.V. catheter removal

- A peripheral I.V. line is removed on completion of therapy, for cannula site changes, and for suspected infection, thrombophlebitis, or infiltration.

The write stuff

- After removing an I.V. line, document the date and time of removal.
- Describe the condition of the site.
- If drainage was present at the puncture site, document that you sent the tip of the device and a sample of the drainage to the laboratory for culture, according to your facility's policy.
- Record any site care given and the type of dressing applied.
- Document any patient instructions provided.

| 10/15/06 | 1000 | I.V. catheter removed from ® forearm vein. Pressure held for 2 min. until bleeding stopped. Site clean and dry, no redness, drainage, warmth, or pain noted. Dry sterile dressing applied to site. Pt. instructed to call nurse if bleeding, swelling, redness, or pain occurs at the removal site. —— Alexis Karev, RN |

I.V. site care

- Proper I.V. site care is the single most important intervention for preventing infection and other complications.
- Typically, I.V. dressings are changed every 48 hours or whenever the dressing becomes wet, soiled, or nonocclusive.
- The site should be assessed:
  - routinely if a transparent semipermeable dressing is used
  - with dressing changes if another type of dressing is used.
- Check your facility's policy for frequency of I.V. dressing changes and the type of site care to be performed.

The write stuff

- In your notes or on the appropriate I.V. sheets, record the date and time of the dressing change.
- Chart the condition of the insertion site, noting whether there are signs of:
  - infection (redness and pain)
  - infiltration (coolness, blanching, and edema)
  - thrombophlebitis (redness, firmness, pain along the path of the vein, and edema).
- If complications occur, note:
  - name of the practitioner notified and time of notification
  - orders received
  - your interventions and the patient's response to them.
- Record site care given and the type of dressing applied.
- Document patient education provided.

12/02/06	0910	Transparent I.V. dressing wet and curling at
		edges. Dressing removed. Skin cleaned with
		alcohol, air dried. No redness, blanching,
		warmth, coolness, edema, drainage, or
		induration noted. No c/o pain at site. New
		transparent dressing applied and secured with
		tape. Pt. told to report any pain at site.
		———— Catherine Willows, RN

I.V. site change

- Routine maintenance of an I.V. site and rotation of the site help prevent complications, such as thrombophlebitis and infection.
- The I.V. site is changed every 48 to 72 hours, according to your facility's policy.
- An I.V. site that shows signs of infection, infiltration, or thrombophlebitis should be changed immediately.

The write stuff

- In your note or on the appropriate I.V. sheets, record the date and time that the I.V. line was removed.
- Note whether the site change is routine or due to a complication.
- Describe the condition of the site.
- Record site care given and the type of dressing applied.
- Document the new I.V. insertion site.
- Record the type, gauge, and length of the needle or catheter.
- Include the number of attempts at venipuncture, if you made more than one.
- Document:
  - type and flow rate of the I.V. solution
  - name and amount of medication in the solution (if any)
  - any adverse effects and actions taken to correct them.
- Record patient education provided.

09/02/06	0900	I.V. line in place for 72 hours and removed from ® forearm according to facility policy. Site without redness, warmth, swelling, or pain. 2" x 2" gauze dressing applied. I.V. infusion restarted in ℚ forearm using 20G 1¹/2" catheter on first attempt. Site dressed with transparent dressing. 500 ml of NSS infusing at 50 ml/hr. Pt. instructed to call nurse immediately for any pain at I.V. site. ———— Chris Jordan, R.N

I.V. site infiltration

- Infiltration occurs when an I.V. solution enters the surrounding tissue as a result of a punctured vein or leakage around a venipuncture site.
- If vesicant drugs or fluids infiltrate, severe local tissue damage may result.
  - Many malpractice cases are brought annually because of the severe nerve and tissue damage from infiltrated I.V. sites that nurses failed to monitor.
  - In some cases, amputations have been necessary because of the nerve and tissue damage.
- Because infiltration can occur without pain or in unresponsive patients, the I.V. site must be monitored frequently.
- Documenting I.V. site assessments and the site care provided is important in preventing and detecting infiltration and other complications.

The write stuff

- Record the date and time of your entry.
- Record signs and symptoms of infiltration at the I.V. site, such as:
  - swelling, burning, discomfort, or pain
  - tight feeling
  - decreased skin temperature
  - blanching.
- Chart your assessment of circulation to the affected and unaffected limbs, such as skin color, capillary refill, pulses, and circumference.
- Estimate the amount of fluid infiltrated.
- Record:
  - name of the practitioner notified
  - time of notification
  - orders received (such as vesicant antidotes, limb elevation, and ice or warm soaks)

- your actions
- patient's response to interventions.
- Note the new I.V. site.
- Record emotional support and patient education provided.

02/10/06	1840	I.V. site in ℞ forearm swollen and cool at
		1820. Pt. c/o of some discomfort at the site.
		Hands warm with capillary refill less than 3
		seconds, strong radial pulses bilaterally. ℞
		forearm circumference 9¹/₂", Ⓛ forearm
		circumference 9". I.V. line removed and
		sterile gauze dressing applied. Approx. 30 ml
		of NSS infiltrated. Dr. Summers notified of
		findings at 1830, and orders given that I.V.
		therapy may be discontinued. ℞ arm elevated
		on 2 pillows and ice applied in wrapped towel
		for 20 min. After ice application, skin cool,
		intact. No c/o burning or numbness. Explained
		importance of keeping arm elevated and to
		call nurse immediately for any pain, burning,
		numbness in ℞ forearm. —— Jackie Tripper, RN

I.V. therapy

- Whether providing fluid or electrolyte replacement, total parenteral nutrition, drugs, or blood products, you'll need to carefully document all facets of I.V. therapy—including administration and any subsequent complications of I.V. therapy.
- An accurate description of your care provides a clear record of treatments and drugs received by your patient.
- This record provides:
  - legal protection for you and your employer
  - health care insurers with the data they need to approve and provide reimbursement for equipment and supplies.

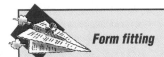

Form fitting

I.V. flow sheet

This sample shows the features of an I.V. flow sheet.

INTRAVENOUS CARE RECORD

Patient's name: _Jennifer Lopen_   Medical record #: _236541_

Intravenous care comment codes: **C** = cap   **F** = filter   **T** = tubing   **D** = dressing

Start date/time	Initials	I.V. volume and solution	Additives	Flow rate	Site
06/30/06 1100	DM	1000 ml D₅W	20 mEq KCL	100/hr	RF A
06/30/06 2100	JS	1000 ml D₅W	20 mEq KCL	100/hr	RF A
07/01/06 0700	DM	1000 ml D₅W	20 mEq KCL	100/hr	LF A

- Depending on your facility's policy, you'll document I.V. therapy on a special I.V. therapy sheet, nursing flow sheet, or other format.

The write stuff

- On each shift:
  - document the type, amount, and flow rate of I.V. fluid
  - condition of the I.V. site.
- Chart each time you flush the I.V. line, and identify any drug used to flush the line.
- Document any change in routine care, along with follow-up assessments.
- Record patient teaching that you perform with the patient and his family.

Stop date/time	Tubing change	Comments/assessment of site
06/30/06 2100	T	
07/01/06 0700		
07/02/06	TD	

L

Late documentation

- Late documentation entries are appropriate in some situations:
  - if the chart was unavailable when it was needed—for example, when the patient was away from the unit
  - if you need to add important information after completing your notes
  - if you forgot to write notes on a particular chart.
- A late or altered chart entry can arouse suspicions and can be a significant problem in the event of a malpractice lawsuit.
- If you must make a late entry or alter an entry, find out if your facility has a protocol for doing so.

The write stuff

- Add the entry to the first available line, and label it "late entry" to indicate that it's out of sequence, according to facility policy.
- Record the date and time of the entry and, in the body of the entry, record the date and time it should have been made.

| 12/25/06 | 0900 Late entry | (Chart not available 12/24/06 at 1500; pt. was in radiology) On 12/13/06 at 1300, pt. stated she felt faint when getting OOB on 12/13/06 at 1200 and she fell to the floor. Pt. states, "The fall didn't hurt at the time, so I didn't think I needed to tell anyone. My husband said I should say something." ® wrist bruised and slightly swollen. Pt. c/o some tenderness. Dr. Kringle notified of pt.'s statement at 1310 and came to see pt. at 1320 on 12/24/06. X-ray of wrist ordered. —— Elaine Kasmer, RN |

Making a case

Documenting late entries

If the court uncovers alterations in a patient's chart during the course of a trial, suspicions may be aroused. The court may infer that additional alterations were made. In such situations, the value of the entire medical record may be brought into question.

Case in point

In one case, the nurse failed to chart her observations of a patient for 7 hours after a surgery, during which time the patient died. The patient's family sued the hospital, charging the nurse with malpractice. The nurse insisted that she had observed the patient but, because her particular unit was understaffed and overpopulated, she wasn't able to record her observations. She explained that the assistant director of nursing later instructed her about the hospital's policy on charting late additions. The nurse subsequently added her observations to the patient's medical record.

Judgment day

Despite the addition of the late entries, the court wasn't convinced that the nurse had observed the patient during the postoperative period. Suspicious of the altered record, it ruled that the nurse's failure to chart her observations at the proper time supported the plaintiff's claim that she had made no such observations.

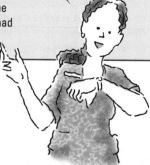

Latex hypersensitivity

- Latex, derived from the sap of the rubber tree, is used throughout the health care industry.
- If your patient has latex hypersensitivity, use only latex-free products.
- Be prepared to treat life-threatening hypersensitivity with antihistamines, epinephrine, corticosteroids, I.V. fluids, oxygen, intubation, and mechanical ventilation, if necessary.
- Alert the pharmacy and other departments that the patient has a latex allergy so that latex-free materials can be provided.
- Place a band on the patient's wrist and on the medical record to identify the hypersensitivity to latex.

The write stuff

- Record the date and time of your entry.
- On admission, record all allergies, including reactions to latex.
- Document signs and symptoms that you observe or that the patient reports to you, such as red skin, itching, hives, wheezing, bronchospasm, or laryngeal edema.
- Include information about diagnostic testing the patient may undergo to confirm latex hypersensitivity.
- Document that other departments have been notified of the patient's latex allergy and that identification of this allergy has been placed on the patient's wrist and on the front of the medical record.
- Describe measures taken to prevent latex exposure.
- Document any patient teaching provided about latex reactions.

| 03/31/06 | 1120 | Pt. reports that she has a latex allergy and has developed red skin and itching with past exposures to latex. Latex allergy wristband placed on pt.'s Ⓛ wrist. Latex precautions stickers placed on pt.'s medical record, MAR, nursing Kardex, and door to pt.'s room. Pharmacy, dietary, lab, and other departments notified of latex allergy by automated record-keeping system. Supply cart with latex-free products kept by pt.'s room. Pt. very knowledgeable about her latex allergy and was able to describe s/s of reactions, products to avoid, and how to respond to a reaction with autoinjectable epinephrine, if necessary. Pt. already sent away for an ID bracelet to identify her latex allergy, but she hasn't yet received it. ——————————— Dawn Knotts, RN |

Level of consciousness

- A patient's level of consciousness (LOC) provides information about his level of responsiveness and neurologic status.
- The Glasgow Coma Scale provides a standard reference for assessing or monitoring the LOC of a patient with a suspected or confirmed brain injury.

The write stuff

- Record the date and time of your assessment.
- Depending on your facility's Glasgow Coma Scale flow sheet, you'll either circle the number that describes your patient's response to stimuli or you'll write in the number of the corresponding response.
- Record the total of the three types of responses.
- If your patient's LOC deteriorates, your narrative note should include:
  - date and time of the entry
  - Glasgow Coma Scale scores and times they were obtained
  - results of your neurologic and vital signs assessments
  - name of the practitioner notified
  - time of notification
  - orders received
  - your interventions
  - patient's response to interventions.
- Chart any patient or family education you gave.

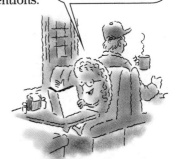

When your patient's neurologic status is in question, the Glasgow Coma Scale is on the menu.

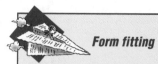

Form fitting

Using the Glasgow Coma Scale

The Glasgow Coma Scale is a standard reference that's used to assess or monitor level of consciousness in a patient with a suspected or confirmed brain injury. This scale measures three responses to stimuli—eye opening response, motor response, and verbal response—and assigns a number to each of the possible responses within these categories. The lowest possible score is 3; the highest is 15. A score of 7 or lower indicates coma. This scale is commonly used in the emergency department, at the scene of an accident, and for the evaluation of a hospitalized patient.

GLASGOW COMA SCALE

Patient name: _John Gladstone_   MR#: _123456_

Characteristic	Response	Score
	Date/time	03/23/06 2000
Eye opening response	• Spontaneous	4
	• To verbal command	③
	• To pain	2
	• No response	1
Best motor response	• Obeys commands	⑥
	• To painful stimulus:	
	– Localizes pain; pushes stimulus away	5
	– Flexes and withdraws	4
	– Abnormal flexion	3
	– Extension	2
	– No response	1
Best verbal response (arouse patient with painful stimulus, if necessary)	• Oriented and converses	5
	• Disoriented and converses	④
	• Uses inappropriate words	3
	• Makes incomprehensible sounds	2
	• No response	1
	Total:	13

03/24/06	0900	Went in pt.'s room with his breakfast at 0830.
		His speech was slurred. Glasgow Coma Scale 11,
		down from 13 at 0600. See Glasgow Coma
		Scale flow sheet for frequent assessments.
		Patient is opening eyes to verbal commands,
		obeys simple commands. PERRLA. ® hand grasp
		is strong, Ⓛ hand grasp is weak. Ⓛ eyelid and
		side of mouth drooping. P 88 reg, RR 24, BP
		122/84, axillary temp 97.2° F. Skin warm, dry.
		Peripheral pulses strong and palpable. Lungs
		clear, normal heart sounds. Dr. Hunt notified
		of change in Glasgow Coma Scale score and
		assessment findings at 0835 and came to see
		pt. at 0840. Patient placed on O₂ at 2 L by
		NC. I.V. infusion of NSS at KVO rate started
		in Ⓛ forearm with 18G catheter. Dr. Hunt
		called pt.'s wife at 0845 to alert her to
		husband's change in LOC. Wife gave consent
		for CT scan. ————————— Mary O'Leary, RN

Life support termination

- According to the right-to-die laws of most states, a patient has the right to refuse extraordinary life-supporting measures if he has no hope of recovery.
- If the patient can't make this decision, advance directives are implemented or the patient's next of kin may be permitted to decide if life support should continue; however, a written statement of the patient's wishes is always preferable.
- If life support is to be terminated:
– read the patient's advance directive to ensure that the present situation matches the patient's wishes
– verify that the risk manager has reviewed the advance directive.
- Check that the appropriate consent forms have been signed.
- Ask the patient's family whether they would like to:
  – see the chaplain
  – be with the patient before, during, and after life support termination.

The write stuff

- Record the date and time of your entry.
- Document whether an advance directive is present and whether it matches your patient's present situation and life support wishes.
- Note that your facility's risk manager has reviewed the advance directive.
- Document that a consent form has been signed to terminate life support, according to facility policy.

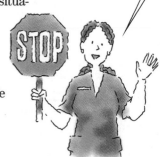

Before terminating life support, have the risk manager review the patient's advance directive.

- Document the names of persons who were notified of the decision to terminate life support and their responses.
- Describe physical care for the patient before and after life-support termination.
- Note whether the family was with the patient before, during, and after termination of life support.
- Record whether a chaplain was present.
- Document the time of termination, name of the practitioner who turned off the equipment, and names of people present.
- Record vital signs after extubation as well as the time the patient stopped breathing, the time he was pronounced dead, and who made the pronouncement.
- Document:
  - family's response
  - your interventions for them
  - postmortem care for the patient.

| 02/28/06 | 1800 | Advance directive provided by pt.'s wife Linda Jones. Document reviewed by risk manager, Michael Scott, who verified that it matched the pt.'s present situation. Wife signed consent form to terminate life support. Wife spent approx. 10 min. alone with pt. before termination of life support. Declined to have anyone with her during this time. Life support terminated at 1730 by Dr. Halpert, with myself, Chaplain Schrute, and pt.'s wife present. VS after extubation: P 50, BP 50/20, no respiratory effort noted. Pronounced dead at 1737. Pt.'s wife tearful. Chaplain Schrute and myself stayed with her and listened to her talk about her 35 years with her husband. Pt. bathed and dressed in pajamas for family visitation. ———————— Pam Beesley, RN |

Lumbar puncture

- Lumbar puncture involves the insertion of a sterile needle into the subarachnoid space of the spinal canal, usually between the third and fourth lumbar vertebrae.
- It's used to:
  - examine cerebrospinal fluid (CSF)
  - measure CSF pressure
  - detect presence of blood in CSF
  - obtain CSF specimens for laboratory analysis
  - inject dyes or gases for contrast in radiologic studies
  - administer drugs, including anesthetics
  - decrease CSF pressure in some instances.

The write stuff

- Record the date and time of your entry.
- Document that the patient understands the procedure and has signed a consent form.
- Record your patient teaching about what to expect before, during, and after the procedure.
- Record the start and completion times of the procedure.
- Document adverse reactions, such as changes in level of consciousness or vital signs and dizziness.
- Chart that you reported adverse reactions to the practitioner and note his response, orders received, your actions, and the patient's response.
- Record the:
  - number of test tube specimens of CSF that were collected
  - time they were transported to the laboratory.
- Describe the color, consistency, and other characteristics of the collected specimens.
- Document the patient's tolerance of the procedure.

- After the procedure, document your interventions, such as:
  - keeping the patient flat in bed for 6 to 12 hours
  - encouraging fluid intake
  - assessing for headache
  - checking the puncture site for leakage of CSF.
- Record the patient's responses to interventions.

10/08/06	0900	Lumbar puncture explained to pt. by Dr.
		Dorian. Pt. verbalized understanding of the
		procedure and signed consent form. Explained
		what to expect before, during, and after the
		procedure and answered his questions. Pt.
		positioned on Ⓛ side for lumbar puncture. Pt.
		draped and prepped by Dr. Dorian. Specimen
		obtained by Dr. on first attempt. One test tube
		obtained and sent to lab. Specimen clear and
		straw colored. Preprocedure, 0815, P 88,
		BP 126/82, RR 18, oral T 98.2° F. During pro-
		cedure, 0830, P 92, BP 128/80, RR 18. After
		procedure, 0845, P 86, BP 132/82, RR 20, oral
		T 98.0° F. Pt. maintained in supine position as
		instructed. I.V. of NSS infusing at 100 ml/hr
		in Ⓡ forearm. Puncture site dressed by Dr.
		Dorian. Site clear, dry, and intact. No leakage.
		Pt. has no c/o of headache or dizziness. Pt.
		reports no pain after procedure. Pt. lying flat
		in bed without difficulty. Pt. drank 240 ml
		ginger ale. ———————— Elliot Reed, RN

M

Mechanical ventilation

- A mechanical ventilator moves air in and out of a patient's lungs.
- *Positive-pressure ventilators* exert a positive pressure on the airway, causing inspiration and increasing tidal volume.
- A *high-frequency ventilator* uses high respiratory rates and low tidal volume to maintain alveolar ventilation.
- *Negative-pressure ventilators*, such as the iron lung, cuirass (chest shell), and body wrap, create negative pressure, which pulls the thorax outward and allows air to flow into the lungs.

The write stuff

- Record the date and time of your entry.
- Note the type of ventilator and its settings, such as:
  - ventilatory mode
  - tidal volume
  - rate
  - fraction of inspired oxygen
  - positive end-expiratory pressure
  - peak inspiratory flow.
- Record:
  - size of the endotracheal (ET) tube
  - centimeter mark of the ET tube
  - cuff pressure.
- Document the patient's:
  - vital signs
  - breath sounds
  - use of accessory muscles
  - comfort level
  - physical appearance.

I don't want to make any waves with my charting, so I'd better document this tidal volume.

- Document complications that occur as well as:
  - name of the practitioner notified and time of notification
  - orders received
  - your interventions
  - patient's response to interventions.
- Record pertinent laboratory data, including arterial blood gas analyses and oxygen saturation findings.
- Record tracheal suctioning and the character of secretions.
- If the patient is receiving pressure-support ventilation or is using a T piece or tracheostomy collar, note:
  - duration of spontaneous breathing
  - patient's ability to maintain the weaning schedule.
- If the patient is receiving intermittent mandatory ventilation, record:
  - control breath rate
  - rate of spontaneous respirations.
- Record adjustments made in ventilator settings and the patient's response.
- Document ventilator maintenance, such as draining condensate and changing or cleaning the tubing.
- Record patient teaching and emotional support given.

06/16/06	1015	Pt. on Servo ventilator set at TV 750, F$_{IO_2}$ 45%, 5 cm PEEP, Assist-control mode of 12. RR 20 and nonlabored; no SOB or use of accessory muscles noted. #8 ET tube in ℞ corner of mouth taped securely at 22-cm mark. Suctioned via ET tube for large amt. of thick white secretions. Pulse oximetry reading 98%. Ⓛ lung clear. ℞ lung with basilar crackles and expiratory wheezes. Dr. Owens notified of assessment findings at 1000; no treatment at this time. Explained all procedures including suctioning to pt. Pt. nodded head "yes" when asked if he understood explanations. ————————————————— Lucas Wilson, RN

Medication error

- Medication errors are the most common, and potentially the most dangerous, nursing errors.
- Mistakes in dosage, administration route, patient identification, or drug selection by nurses have led to vision loss, brain damage, cardiac arrest, and death.
- A medication event report or incident report should be completed when a medication error is discovered.
- The nurse who discovers the medication error is responsible for completing the medication event report or incident report and for communicating the error to the patient's practitioner and the nursing supervisor.

Making a case

Lawsuits and medication errors

Unfortunately, lawsuits involving nurses' drug errors are common. The court determines liability based on the standards of care required of nurses who administer drugs. In many instances, if the nurse had known more about the proper dosage, administration route, or procedure connected with a drug's use, she might have avoided the mistake.

Case in point
In *Norton v. Argonaut Insurance Co.* (1962), an infant died after a nurse administered injectable digoxin at a dosage level appropriate for elixir of Lanoxin, an oral drug. The nurse was unaware that digoxin was available in an oral form. The nurse questioned two doctors who weren't treating the infant about the order but failed to mention to them that the order was written for elixir of Lanoxin. She also failed to clarify the order with the doctor who wrote it.

Judgment day
The nurse, the doctor who ordered the drug, and the hospital were found liable.

- Document the error objectively, avoiding such terms as "by mistake," "somehow," "unintentionally," "miscalculated," and "confusing," which can be interpreted as admissions of wrongdoing.

The write stuff

- Record the date and time of your entry.
- In your nurse's note, describe the situation objectively.
- Include:
  - name of the practitioner notified
  - time of notification
  - orders received
  - your interventions
  - patient's response to interventions.
- Document the medication error on an incident report or medication event report.

10/08/06	1315	Pt. was given Demerol 100 mg I.M. at 1300
		for abdominal pain. Dr. Kelso called at 1305
		and is on his way to see pt. P 80, BP 120/82,
		RR 20, oral T 98.4° F. Alert and oriented to
		time, place, and person. ———— Terry Cox, RN

Form fitting

Medication event quality review form

QUALITY REVIEW FORM

Confidential — This is a peer review document and may be protected by applicable law. Not for distribution.

Patient name: _Jack Dunn_
Medical record #: _555121_

EVENT DATA

Date and time of event: _10/08/06 1300_
Date and time reported: _10/08/06 1315_

Primary event type
(check one only):

- ☐ Wrong drug
- ☐ Wrong dose
- ☐ Omitted dose
- ☑ Wrong time
- ☐ Wrong route
- ☐ Wrong patient
- ☐ Other _____

For wrong dose or omitted doses, # doses involved: _____

Event severity
(check one only):

- ☐ 0 – potential error only
- ☐ 1 – error occurred, no harm to the patient
- ☑ 2 – error occurred, increased monitoring only
- ☐ 3 – error occurred, change in VS, additional labs, no permanent harm
- ☐ 4 – error occurred, required additional treatment, increased LOS
- ☐ 5 – error occurred, permanent harm to patient
- ☐ 6 – error resulted in patient's death

CONTRIBUTING CAUSES OF EVENT

Order related (check all that apply):

Type of order: ☐ Written   ☐ Oral   ☐ Telephone

- ☐ Order incomplete:
  - ☐ Not dated
  - ☐ Not timed
  - ☐ No dose
  - ☐ No route
  - ☐ No frequency
  - ☐ No signature
  - ☐ Signature illegible
  - ☐ No drug parameters indicated
- ☐ Order illegible
- ☐ Unacceptable abbreviation: _____
- ☐ Decimal misplaced
- ☐ Inappropriate use of leading or trailing zeros

- ☐ Order not flagged correctly
- ☐ Order written on wrong patient's chart
- ☐ Inappropriate drug selection
- ☐ Inappropriate route selection
- ☐ Patient drug allergies not identified or documented
- ☐ Drug not renewed
- ☐ Drug not discontinued
- ☐ Drug not reordered postop
- ☐ Nonformulary request

(continued)

Medication event quality review form *(continued)*

Transcription related (check all that apply):
- ☐ Order not faxed
- ☐ Order not transcribed
- ☐ Pharmacy clarification of order not transcribed
- ☐ Incomplete order not clarified
- ☐ Order not completely signed off
- ☐ Incorrect transcription onto:
  - ☐ Not dated ☐ Recopied MAR
- ☐ Transcription illegible on:
  - ☐ MAR ☐ Recopied MAR
- ☐ Incomplete allergy documentation
- ☐ Allergies not transcribed onto:
  - ☐ Order sheets ☐ MAR
  - ☐ Recopied MAR
- ☐ Unacceptable abbreviations

Patient related (check all that apply):
- ☐ Took own meds
- ☐ Altered infusion rate
- ☐ Loss of venous access
- ☐ Medication refused

Dispensing related (check all that apply):
- ☐ Drug incompatibility
- ☐ Outdated product dispensed
- ☐ Patient allergies not identified
- ☐ Incorrect product chosen
- ☐ Product incorrectly labeled
- ☐ Product not delivered to nursing unit
- ☐ Delay in delivery due to:
  - ☐ Nonformulary request
  - ☐ Illegible order
  - ☐ Out of stock
  - ☐ Illegible fax
  - ☐ Further investigation required
  - ☐ Pneumatic tube problem
  - ☐ Other: _____
- ☐ Product incorrectly prepared in:
  - ☐ Pharmacy ☐ Nursing unit
  - ☐ Other: _____
- ☐ Miscalculation
- ☐ No physician order
- ☐ Incomplete physician order not clarified
- ☐ Unacceptable abbreviation: _____
- ☐ Computer entry errors (pharmacy only):
  - ☐ Duplicate ☐ Wrong patient
  - ☐ Missed order ☐ Wrong drug
  - ☐ Other: _____
- ☐ Pharmacy clarification of order not documented

Medication event quality review form *(continued)*

Administration related (check all that apply):

☐ Incorrect drug storage method

☐ Patient allergies not correctly checked against:
   ☐ Allergy band   ☐ MAR

☐ Patient allergy band not intact

☐ Patient not correctly identified

☐ No physician order

☐ Drug incompatibility

☐ Available product incorrectly prepared

☐ Miscalculation

☐ Incorrectly labeled

☐ Medication or I.V. not checked with MAR, order, I.V. record

☑ Time of last p.r.n. medication administration not checked

☐ Patient not observed taking medication

☐ Med. or I.V. not charted at time of administration

☐ Med. or I.V. not charted correctly

☐ Incorrect I.V. line used

☐ Incorrect setting on infusion pump

☐ Lock-out on infusion pump not used

☐ Outdated product given

☐ Forgotten or overlooked

☐ Product not available

☐ Extra or duplicated dose

☐ Monitoring, insufficient or not done

EVENT ANALYSIS

(Include additional information, such as staffing patterns, activity level, patient outcome, action plan, and conclusion)

Carla Espinosa, RN, had administered and documented giving p.r.n. Demerol 100 mg I.M. to the pt. at 1215. I did not review the p.r.n. MAR and administered the dose again at 1300. Pt. monitored q 15 min. for 2 hours. No adverse effects. Pt. alert and oriented to time, place, and person. Dr. Kelso called at 1305 and came to see pt.

Completed by: *Terry Cox, RN*   Date completed: *10/8/06*

Moderate sedation

- Moderate sedation produces a minimally depressed level of consciousness (LOC) in patients undergoing tests; minor surgical procedures, such as minor bone fracture reduction, breast biopsy, vasectomy, and dental or plastic reconstructive surgery; endoscopic procedures; or interventional radiology procedures.
- Moderate sedation allows the patient to respond to verbal or tactile commands and maintain airway patency and protective reflexes while controlling anxiety and pain and producing amnesia.
- The patient is able to return to daily activities within a short time of moderate sedation.
- Drugs, such as benzodiazepines and opioids, may be used alone or in combination to produce moderate sedation.
- Emergency equipment, reversal drugs, and staff trained in advanced cardiac life support must be immediately available for the patient who slips into a deeper level of sedation.
- Know whether your state board of nursing and your facility allow you to administer drugs for moderate sedation.

The write stuff

- Record the date and time of your entry.
- Note the time you received the patient.
- Chart your assessment of the patient's respiratory and cardiovascular assessments, LOC, and vital signs.
- Describe the surgical or procedural site, including:
  – drainage (amount, color, consistency)
  – bleeding
  – swelling
  – condition of skin around the site
  – presence and condition of any dressings or drains.
- Document the patient's level of pain, using a 0-to-10 scale (with 10 being the worst pain imaginable), analgesics or comfort measures given, and the patient's response.

- Flow sheets may be used to record your frequent assessments, vital signs, intake and output, I.V. therapy, sedation level, and neurologic assessments.
- Document any drugs given on the appropriate form; include the patient's response.
- If you detect changes in the patient's condition, such as somnolence, confusion, respiratory depression or obstruction, nausea or vomiting, hypotension, or coma, document:
  – your interventions
  – name of the practitioner notified and orders received
  – patient's response to interventions.
- If the patient is being discharged, note:
  – that discharge criteria were met
  – your discharge instructions
  – who's taking the patient home.
- Document patient and family education and support given.

01/14/06	1300	Received pt. from endoscopy at 1230 via wheel-chair after colonoscopy. P 82 reg, BP 128/72, RR 16 deep, oral T 98.8° F. Pt. awake, alert, and oriented to time, place, and person. Breath sounds clear bilaterally, skin pink, pulse ox. 98% on room air. Peripheral pulses strong and capillary refill brisk. Pt. moving all extremities and able to feel light touch. Cough and gag reflexes intact. Abdomen slightly distended, + bowel sounds X4. Pt. reports some abdominal discomfort but denies the need for any medication. I.V. of 1000 ml NSS infusing at 30 ml/hr in ℗ hand via infusion pump. See flow sheets for frequent V.S., I.V. therapy, I/O, and neuro assessments. Explained to pt. that he may be discharged when he is able to urinate and drink fluids. Pt. given 120 ml of apple juice to sip. He requested that discharge instructions be given to his wife. —————— Marilyn Stokes, RN

Multiple trauma

- The patient with multiple trauma has injuries to more than one body system caused by such situations as vehicular accident, violence, a fall, or a burn.
- Injuries may involve penetrating wounds, blunt trauma, or both.
- Immediately upon arrival at the health care facility, the patient will undergo a primary survey of airway, breathing, and circulation, which includes resuscitation and treatment of life-threatening problems as needed.
- When life-threatening problems are stabilized, a secondary survey is performed.

The write stuff

- On admission, record your primary survey, including:
  - date and time that the patient is admitted to the facility,
  - assessment of airway, breathing, and circulation (including hemorrhage)
  - resuscitation and emergency treatment performed, such as cardiopulmonary resuscitation, intubation, mechanical ventilation, oxygen therapy, fluid or blood replacement, and direct pressure to bleeding
  - patient's level of consciousness.
- When the primary survey is complete, document a more thorough secondary survey, including:
  - cause and physical evidence of trauma
  - vital signs
  - head-to-toe assessment
  - history, including history obtained from family members or others
  - diagnostic tests performed.
- Record treatments provided, such as:
  - insertion of a nasogastric, urinary, or chest tube
  - neck and spine stabilization
  - drug therapy

- splinting of fractures
- wound care.
- Include patient and family teaching and emotional support provided.
- Continue to document ongoing frequent assessments and treatments until the patient's condition has stabilized.
- A critical care or trauma flow sheet may be used.

| 08/15/06 | 1330 | 18 y.o. male brought to ED after being struck by a car at 1245 while riding his bike. Pt. was wearing a helmet. Parents are present. Pt. is awake, alert, and oriented to person and place but not time. Pt. has trauma to face, airway is open, no stridor, RR 18 and nonlabored. Administering O_2 2 L/min by NC. Cervical spine immobilized. P 104, BP 90/62. Monitor shows sinus tachycardia, no arrhythmias. Bruising over abdomen. Pt. splinting abdomen and c/o abdominal pain. Is nauseated but no vomiting. #16 Fr Foley catheter placed at 1255; no blood in urine. I.V. line started with first attempt at 1250 in ® antecubital vein with 18G catheter. 1000 ml of lactated Ringer's infusing at 250 ml/hr. X-rays of neck, spine, and pelvis done at 1315; results pending. Pt. moving upper extremities spontaneously and without pain. Moving Ⓛ leg on own, without pain, ® thigh has bruising and deformity, c/o of ® thigh pain. Radial pulses palpable. Dorsalis pedis and posterior tibial pulses palpable and weak. Able to feel light touch to both legs. Dr. Dobler discussing need for exploratory abdominal surgery and reduction of ® thigh fracture with parents. See I.V., I/O, and VS flow sheets for frequent assessments. Explaining all procedures to pt., allowing parents to be with pt. ————— |
| | | ————————— Carrie Grant, R.N |

Myocardial infarction

- Myocardial infarction (MI) is an occlusion of a coronary artery that leads to oxygen deprivation, myocardial ischemia and, if untreated, necrosis (death of tissue).
- The extent of functional impairment depends on:
  - early intervention
  - size and location of the infarct
  - condition of the uninvolved myocardium
  - potential for collateral circulation
  - effectiveness of compensatory mechanisms.
- Prompt recognition of MI and nursing interventions to relieve chest pain, stabilize heart rhythm, reduce cardiac workload, and revascularize the coronary artery are essential to preserving myocardial tissue and preventing complications, including death.
- Expect to:
  - assist with thrombolytic therapy
  - administer oxygen
  - administer drugs to relieve pain, treat arrhythmias, reduce myocardial oxygen demands, increase myocardial oxygen supply, and improve the patient's chance of survival
  - assist with the insertion of hemodynamic monitoring catheters
  - prepare the patient for invasive procedures to improve coronary circulation.

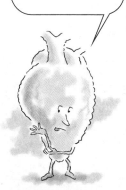

Prompt recognition of MI and interventions to relieve it are essential. So is prompt documentation after the patient has been stabilized.

The write stuff

- Record the date and time of your entry.
- Describe your patient's chest pain and other symptoms of MI, using his words whenever possible.
- Record your assessment findings, such as:
  - feelings of impending doom, anxiety, and restlessness
  - nausea and vomiting
  - dyspnea or tachypnea
  - cool extremities
  - weak peripheral pulses
  - diaphoresis
  - abnormal heart sounds
  - hypotension or hypertension
  - bradycardia or tachycardia
  - crackles on lung auscultation.
- Document:
  - name of the practitioner notified
  - time of notification
  - orders received, such as transfer to the coronary care unit, continuous cardiac monitoring, supplemental oxygen, 12-lead electrocardiogram, and drug therapy
  - your actions
  - patient's response to therapies.
- Use the appropriate flow sheets to record:
  - intake and output
  - hemodynamic parameters
  - I.V. fluids given
  - drugs administered
  - frequent vital signs.
- Record teaching and emotional support given to the patient and his family.

| 12/30/06 | 2310 | Pt. c/o severe crushing midsternal chest pain with radiation to Ⓛ arm at 2240. Pt. pointed to center of chest and stated, "I feel like I have an elephant on my chest." Rates pain at 9 on a scale of 0 to 10, w/10 being the worst pain imaginable. Pt. is restless in bed and diaphoretic, c/o nausea. P 84 and regular, BP 128/82, RR 24, oral T 98.8° F. Extremities cool, pedal pulses weak, normal heart sounds, breath sounds clear. Dr. Burrows notified of pt.'s chest pain and physical findings at 2245 and came to see pt. and orders given. O₂ started at 2 L by NC. 12-lead ECG obtained; showed ST-segment elevation in anterior leads. Pt. placed on portable cardiac monitor. I.V. line started with first attempt in Ⓛ forearm with 18 G catheter with NSS at 30 ml/hr. Stat cardiac enzymes, troponin, myoglobin, and electrolytes sent to lab at 2255. Nitroglycerin 1/150 gr given SL, 5 minutes apart X3 with no relief. Explaining all procedures to pt., who verbalizes understanding. Assuring her that she's being monitored closely and will be transferred to CCU for closer monitoring and treatment. Dr. Burrows called husband Michael Scoffield and notified him of wife's chest pain and transfer. Report called to CCU at 2255 and given to Veronica Donovan, RN. —————————————————————— Sara Tancredi, RN |

N

Nasogastric tube care

- The most commonly used nasogastric (NG) tubes are the single-lumen Levin tube and the double-lumen Salem sump tube.
- Monitoring the patient with an NG tube involves:
  - checking drainage from the NG tube
  - assessing the patient's GI function
  - verifying correct tube placement
  - irrigating the tube to ensure patency to prevent mucosal damage.

The write stuff

- Record the date and time that care was provided.
- Record confirmation of proper tube placement per facility policy.
- Use an intake and output flow sheet to record:
  - fluids you instill in the NG tube
  - NG output.
- Describe the NG drainage, noting its color, consistency, and odor.
- Describe the condition of the patient's skin, mouth, and nares as well as care provided.
- Document tape changes and skin care you provide.
- Record your assessment of bowel sounds.
- Note patient education and emotional support given.

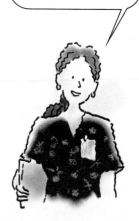

Every NG tube has its place, and you need to confirm and record proper placement.

11/21/06	1100	NG tube placement verified by aspirating 10 ml
		of clear and colorless fluid with mucus shreds
		and pH test strip result of 5. NG tube
		drained 100 ml of clear and colorless fluid
		with mucus shreds over 4 hr. Active bowel
		sounds in all 4 quadrants. Skin around mouth
		and nose intact. Helped pt. brush his teeth
		and rinse mouth, petroleum jelly applied to
		lips, water-soluble lubricant applied to nares.
		Tape secure around nose and not moved at
		this time. Explained importance of good oral
		hygiene to pt. ———— Bud Court, RN

Nasogastric tube insertion

- Usually inserted to decompress the stomach, a nasogastric (NG) tube can prevent vomiting after major surgery or in a patient with a bowel obstruction.
- An NG tube typically remains in place for 48 to 72 hours after surgery and is removed when peristalsis resumes.
- The NG tube has other diagnostic and therapeutic applications, such as:
  - assessing and treating upper GI bleeding
  - collecting gastric contents for analysis
  - performing gastric lavage
  - aspirating gastric secretions
  - administering drugs and nutrients.
- Insertion of an NG tube demands close observation of the patient and verification of proper tube placement.

The write stuff

- Record:
  - type and size of the NG tube inserted
  - date, time, and route of insertion
  - confirmation of proper placement.
- Describe the type and amount of suction.
- Describe the drainage characteristics, such as amount, color, consistency, character, and odor.
- Record the patient's tolerance of the insertion procedure.

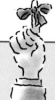

Memory jogger

Documentation of the characteristics of NG tube drainage is nothing to sneeze at. To remember what characteristics to document, think **ACCChO:**

Amount

Color

Consistency

Character

Odor.

- Include signs and symptoms signaling complications, such as nausea, vomiting, and abdominal distention.
- Document subsequent irrigation procedures and continuing problems after irrigations.
- Include patient education and emotional support given.

04/22/06	1700	Procedure explained to pt. by Dr. Grissom. #12 Fr. NG tube inserted via ℗ nostril by Dr. Grissom. Placement verified by aspiration of green stomach contents and pH test strip result of 5. Tube attached to low intermittent suction as ordered. Tube taped in place to nose. Drainage pale green, Hematest negative. Irrigated with 30 ml NSS per order. Hypoactive bowel sounds in all 4 quadrants. Pt. resting comfortably in bed. No c/o nausea or pain. ——————— Sara Sidle, RN

Nasogastric tube removal

- A nasogastric (NG) tube typically remains in place for 48 to 72 hours after surgery and is removed when peristalsis resumes.
- Depending on its use, it may remain in place for shorter or longer periods.

The write stuff

- Record the date and time that the NG tube is removed.
- Document that you have explained the procedure to the patient.
- Describe the color, consistency, and amount of gastric drainage.
- Document the results of your GI assessment.
- Note the patient's tolerance of the procedure.

04/24/06	0900	Explained the procedure of NG tube removal
		to pt. Active bowel sounds heard in all 4
		quadrants No c/o abdominal pain. Drained 25
		ml of pale green odorless drainage over last
		2 hr. Pt. tolerating ice chips without nausea,
		vomiting, discomfort, or abdominal distention.
		NG tube removed without difficulty. Pt. taking
		small sips of water without c/o nausea. Pt.
		stated, "Taking the tube out wasn't as bad as I
		thought." ———————— Sara Sidle, RN

Noncompliance

- Occasionally, a patient is noncompliant, meaning he does something—or fails to do something—that may contribute to an injury or explain why he hasn't responded to nursing and medical care.

The write stuff

- Record the date and time of your entry.
- Document noncompliant patient behaviors and their outcomes.
- Document the name of the practitioner notified and the time of notification.
- Document behavior that runs counter to medical instructions as well as the fact that you informed the patient of the possible consequences of his actions.

08/31/06	0800	Pt. up and walking in hall without antiembolism stockings on. Reminded pt. that stockings need to be put on before getting out of bed, before edema develops, to be most effective. Pt. stated, "It's too early. I'll put them on after breakfast." Dr. Hutchins notified of the situation at 0750. No orders given. Dr. Hutchins will talk with pt. this afternoon. ——————— Casey Martin, R.N

O–Q

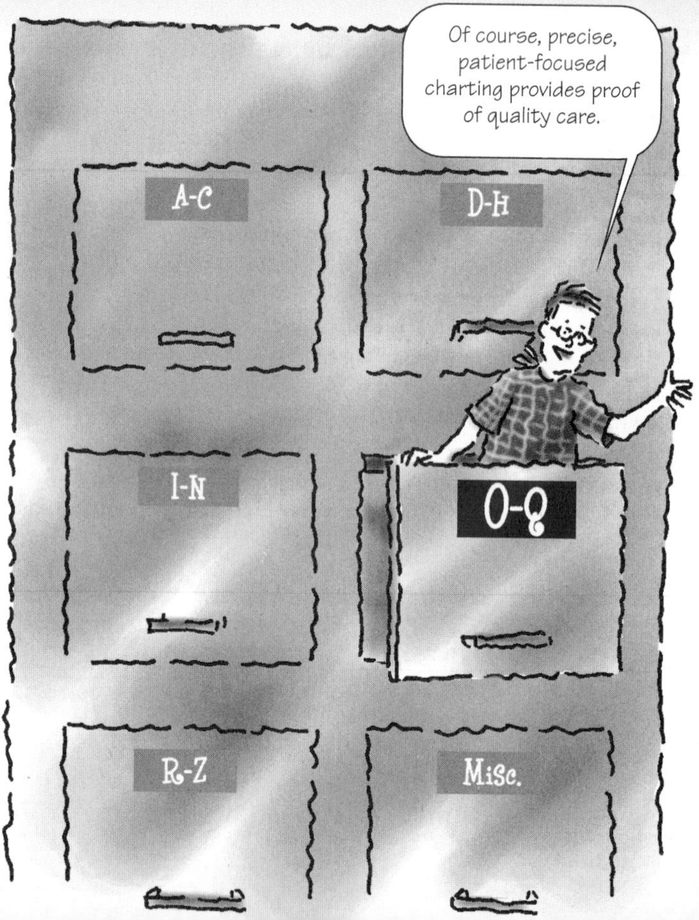
Of course, precise, patient-focused charting provides proof of quality care.
A-C
D-H
I-N
O-Q
R-Z
Misc.

One-time drug administration

- Single-dose medications, which can include a supplemental dose or a stat dose, should be documented in the:
  - one-time medication administration section of the record
  - progress notes.
- When transcribing a one-time order to be given on another shift, be sure to communicate information to the next shift during report, or use a medication alert sticker to flag the order.

The write stuff

- Record the date and time of your entry.
- Include the name of the person who ordered the drug.
- Tell why the order was given.
- Describe the patient's response to the drug.
- Document your assessments to show that you monitored the patient for:
  - adverse effects
  - other potential outcomes
  - changes in condition.
- Use flow sheets, as indicated, to document frequent assessments.

| 06/05/06 | 1100 | Pt. agreed to influenza virus vaccine after Dr. Bryan explained that she was in the high-risk category because of her advanced age and long history of COPD. Dr. Bryan also explained risks of vaccine to pt. Pt. denies allergic reaction to eggs, chicken, or chicken feathers or dander. Pt. is afebrile, oral T 97.2° F, and has no active infections. Fluzone 0.5 ml I.M. injected in Ⓡ deltoid. Explained fever, malaise, and myalgia may occur up to 2 days after vaccination and site may feel tender. Pt verbalized understanding of all teaching. ——— ——————————————————— Tricia Takanawa, RN |

Opioid inventory

- When you administer opioids, you must follow stringent federal, state, and institutional regulations concerning administration and documentation of these drugs.
- An institution is subject to heavy penalties when regulations are breached.
- Government regulations require:
  - opioid drugs to be counted after each nursing shift to ensure an accurate drug count
  - a second nurse to document your activity and observe you if an opioid or part of a dose must be wasted.
- Many facilities use an automated storage system for opioids that eliminates the need for counting the opioids at the end of a shift.
  - This system allows the nurse easy access (via an ID and password or fingerprint) to medications, including other drugs and floor stocks for nursing units.
  - Nurses may remove medications by selecting the patient, medication, and amount needed on the keypad.
  - The nurse must then count the amount of the drug remaining in the system and enter it.
  - Each transaction is recorded and copies are sent to the pharmacy and billing department.

The write stuff

- If not automated, use the special control sheets provided by the pharmacy and follow these procedures:
  - Sign out the drug on the appropriate form.
  - Verify the amount of drug in the container before giving it.
  - Have another nurse document your activity and observe you if you must waste or discard part of an opioid dose.
- At the end of your shift:
  - Record the amount of each opioid on the opioid control sheet while the nurse beginning her shift counts the opioids out loud.

- Sign the opioid control sheet only if the count is correct and have the other nurse countersign.
- Identify and correct any discrepancies before any nurse leaves the unit.
• If a discrepancy can't be resolved, follow your employer's policy for reporting and filing an incident report.

Form fitting

Sample opioid control sheet

The sample opioid control sheet demonstrates proper documentation of opioids and an end-of-shift opioid count.

CITY HOSPITAL
24-hour record
Controlled substances

Unit __45__   Date __01/05/06__

	Codeine 30 mg tab	Percocet tab	Tylenol #3 tab	Valium 2 mg tab	Valium 5 mg tab	Temazepam 15 mg tab	Demerol 50mg inj	Demerol 75mg inj	Demerol 100mg inj	Dilaudid 2 mg inj	Morphine 2mg inj	Morphine 10mg inj	Versed 2ml inj	Dose	Amount wasted	Initials	Witness initials
7 a.m. inventory	25	20	18	15	16	10	10	8	5	10	15	13	3				
Patient name / Pat. no.																	
0915 Orr, Carl 555112												12		5mg	5mg	MS	DB
1000 Davis, Donna 555161		16												ii		MK	
1115 McGowen, John 555111					15									T		KC	

Init.	Signature	Init.	Signature
MS	M Stevens, RN		
MK	M. Keller, RN		
KC	K. Collins, RN		

Organ donation

- A federal requirement enacted in 1998 requires facilities to report deaths to the regional organ procurement organization (OPO) so that no potential donor would be missed.
- The regulation ensures that the family of every potential donor will understand the option to donate.
- Collection of most organs, including the heart, liver, kidney, and pancreas, requires that the patient be pronounced brain dead and kept physically alive until the organs are harvested.
- Tissue, such as eyes, skin, bone, and heart valves, may be taken after death.
- Follow your facility's policy for identifying and reporting a potential organ donor.
- Contact your local or regional OPO when a potential donor is identified.
- A specially trained person from your facility along with someone from your regional OPO will speak with the family about organ donation.
- The OPO coordinates the donation process after a family consents to donation.
- Your documentation will vary depending on the stage of, and your role in, the organ donation process.

The write stuff

- Record the date and time of each note.
- Record the date and time that the patient is pronounced brain dead and the doctor's discussions with the family about the prognosis.
- If the patient's driver's license or other documents indicate his wish to donate organs, place copies in the medical record and document that you have done so.

- The individual who contacts the regional OPO must document the conversation, including:
  - date and time
  - name of the person he spoke with
  - instructions received.
- If you were part of the discussion about organ donation with the family, document:
  - who was present
  - what the family was told and by whom
  - family's response.
- Continue to record your nursing care of the donor until the time he is taken to the operating room for organ procurement.
- Document teaching, explanations, and emotional support given to the family.

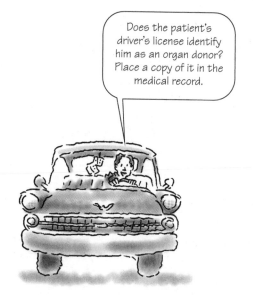

11/12/06	0900	Dr. Shepherd explained at 0815 that pt. was
		brain dead and the prognosis. Mary Bailey,
		wife; George Bailey, son; Clara Stewart,
		daughter; and I were present. Family asked
		about organ donation. Wife stated, "My
		husband had spoken about donating his organs
		if this type of situation ever occurred. I
		believe his driver's license says he's an organ
		donor." Driver's license located with pt.'s
		belongings and removed from wallet by wife.
		License confirms pt.'s request for organ
		donation. Copy of license placed in medical
		record. Dr. Shepherd explained the criteria
		for organ donation and the process to the
		family. Mrs. Bailey stated she would like more
		information from the regional OPO. OPO was
		contacted by this nurse at 0830. Intake
		information was taken by Rhonda Addison.
		Appointment made for today at 1100 for OPO
		coordinator to meet with family in conference
		room on nursing unit. Family also requested
		to speak with a chaplain. Chaplain was paged,
		and Fr. Stone will be here at 0915 to meet
		with family. Family given use of private waiting
		room on the unit for privacy. Checking with
		family every hour to see if there is anything
		they need, to answer questions, and to provide
		support. ———————————— Alex Woods, RN

Ostomy care

- An ostomy is a surgically created opening used to replace a normal physiologic function.
- Ostomies facilitate the elimination of solid or liquid waste or to support respirations if placed in the trachea.
- The type and amount of care an ostomy requires depend on the output and location of the stoma.
- The nurse is responsible for providing ostomy care and assessing the condition of the stoma.
- The nurse may also need to help the patient adapt to the care and wearing of an appliance while helping him accept the body change.

The write stuff

- Record the date and time of ostomy care.
- Describe the:
  - location of the ostomy
  - condition of the stoma, including size, shape, and color.
- Chart the condition of the peristomal skin, noting any redness, irritation, breakdown, bleeding, or other unusual conditions.
- Note the character of drainage, including color, amount, type, and consistency.
- Record:
  - type of appliance used
  - appliance size
  - type of adhesive used.
- Document patient teaching and emotional support given.
- Record the patient's response to teaching and self-care of the ostomy.
- Document the patient's learning progress.

06/11/06	1000	Ostomy located in ① upper abdomen. Appliance removed, minimal amount of dark brown fecal material in bag. Stoma 4 cm in diameter, round, beefy red in color; no drainage or bleeding. Skin surrounding stoma is pink and intact. Karaya ring applied to skin surrounding stoma after applying skin adhesive. New appliance snapped onto ring. Pt. helped measure stoma and applied skin adhesive. Pt. currently reading material on ostomy care and has asked many questions. Discussed proper measurement of stoma and cutting hole in skin barrier to proper size. Pt. understands and agrees to cut skin barrier with next change. Pt. asking many questions about ostomy care. ——————— Marian Payne, RN

Oxygen administration

- A patient needs oxygen therapy when hypoxemia results from a respiratory or cardiac emergency or an increase in metabolic function.
- Signs of hypoxia may include increased heart rate, arrhythmias, restlessness, dyspnea, use of accessory muscles, flared nostrils, cyanosis, decreased level of consciousness (LOC), and cool, clammy skin.
- The adequacy of oxygen therapy is determined by arterial blood gas (ABG) analysis, oximetry monitoring, and clinical assessments.
- The patient's disease, physical condition, and age will help determine the most appropriate method of administration.

The write stuff

- Record your assessment findings, including:
  - vital signs
  - skin color and temperature
  - respiratory effort
  - use of accessory muscles
  - breath sounds
  - LOC.
- Record the date and time of oxygen administration.
- Document the oxygen delivery device used and oxygen flow rate.
- Record ABG or oximetry values.
- If a practitioner was notified, include:
  - name of the practitioner
  - time notified

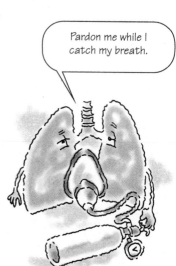

Pardon me while I catch my breath.

- orders received
- whether the practitioner came to see the patient.
• Record the patient's response to oxygen therapy.
• Include any patient teaching and emotional support given.

| 02/16/06 | 1152 | When walking in room at 1130 to bring pt. his lunch tray, noted pt. sitting upright, pale, diaphoretic, taking deep labored breaths using accessory muscles with nasal flaring. O_2 currently at 2 L by nasal cannula. Pt. only able to speak 1-2 words at a time, stated his breathing has been "getting short" over the last hour. P 124 regular, BP 134/88, RR 32 and labored, tymp temp 97.2° F. Skin cool and pale, cyanosis noted around lips. Normal heart sounds, wheezes heard posteriorly on expiration. Pt. alert and oriented to time, place, and person, but appears anxious and restless. Pulse oximetry 87%. Dr. Desmond notified of findings at 1140 and came to see pt. at 1145. Orders given. O_2 increased to 4 L by nasal cannula. Albuterol 2 puffs administered by inhaler. 1145 pt. stated he's "breathing easier." P 92 and regular, BP 128/82, RR 24 and unlabored. Pulse oximetry 96%. No use of accessory muscles noted, skin warm and pink. Lungs clear. Pt. resting comfortably in bed. Explained to pt. the importance of immediately reporting SOB to the nurse. Pt. verbalized understanding. Per orders, O_2 to be titrated to keep O_2 sat greater than 92%. 1150 O_2 sat by pulse oximetry 96%, O_2 reduced back to 2 L. Will recheck O_2 sat in 10 min. —— Libby Widmore, RN |

PQ

Pacemaker (permanent) care

- A pacemaker, implanted when the heart's natural pacemaker fails to work properly, provides electrical impulses to the cardiac muscle to stimulate contraction and support cardiac output.
- Many types of pacemakers are available and most can be programmed to perform various functions.
- Implantable cardioverter defibrillators (ICDs) are commonly placed and may provide the same pacing as a standard pacemaker.
- Know what type of pacemaker the patient has, its rate, and how it works so that you can determine if it's functioning properly and detect complications.
- The patient should have a manufacturer's card with pacemaker information; his medical records may also contain this information.

The write stuff

- Record the date and time of your entry.
- Document:
  - date of pacemaker insertion
  - pacemaker type (demand or fixed rate, defibrillator function)
  - rate of pacing
  - chambers paced
  - chambers sensed
  - how the pulse generator responds
  - whether the pacemaker is rate-responsive.
- Record the three- to five-letter pacemaker code, if known.
- Document the patient's apical pulse rate, noting whether it's regular or irregular.

- If the patient is on a cardiac monitor, place a rhythm strip in the chart, noting the presence of pacemaker spikes, P waves, and QRS complexes and their relationship to each other.
- Record symptoms of pacemaker malfunction, such as dizziness, fainting, weakness, fatigue, chest pain, and prolonged hiccups.
- Document your assessment of the pacemaker insertion site.
- Document any patient education and your patient's understanding of his pacemaker.

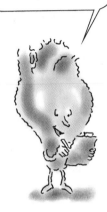

Chart the specs of the pacemaker device used, such as the pacing rate and whether it's rate-responsive.

| 11/24/06 | 1500 | Pt. admitted to unit for treatment of exacerbation of ulcerative colitis. Pt. reports having a permanent DDD pacemaker with low rate set at 60, high rate set at 125, and AV interval of 200 msec. Pacemaker inserted 1998, AP 72 and regular, BP 132/84, RR 18, oral T 97.0° F. Pacemaker site in Ⓡ upper chest w/ healed incision. Pt. denies any dizziness, fainting spells, chest pain, or hiccups. Has been feeling weak and fatigued recently but states he feels this is due to a flare-up of his ulcerative colitis. Pt. able to explain pacemaker function, how to take his pulse, signs and symptoms to report, and need to avoid electromagnetic interference. ————— Thomas Hart, RN |

Pacemaker (permanent) insertion

- A permanent pacemaker is a self-contained unit designed to operate for 3 to 20 years.
- In an operating room or cardiac catheterization laboratory, a surgeon implants the device in a pocket under the patient's skin.
- A permanent pacemaker allows the patient's heart to beat on its own but prevents pacing from falling below a preset rate.
- Pacing electrodes can be placed in the atria, the ventricles, or both.
- Pacemakers may:
  - pace at a rate that varies in response to intrinsic conditions such as skeletal muscle activity
  - have antitachycardia and shock functions.

The write stuff

- Record the date and time of your entry.
- Record the time that the patient returned to your unit.
- Document:
  - type of pacemaker used
  - pacing rate.
- Be sure to include a rhythm strip in your documentation.
- Verify that the chart contains information on the pacemaker's serial number and its manufacturer's name.
- Note whether the pacemaker reduces or eliminates the arrhythmia.
- Describe the condition of the incision site.
- Chart the patient's vital signs and level of consciousness:
  - every 15 minutes for the first hour
  - every hour for the next 4 hours
  - every 4 hours for the next 48 hours
  - once every shift, or according to policy or practitioner's order, thereafter.

- Use a critical care or frequent vital signs flow sheet to document frequent assessments, according to policy.
- Record signs and symptoms of complications, such as infection, lead displacement, perforated ventricle, cardiac tamponade, or lead fracture and disconnection.
- In the event of complications, record:
  - name of the practitioner notified
  - time of notification
  - interventions performed
  - patient's response to interventions.
- Document your patient teaching.

01/28/06	1445	Pt. returned from OR at 1430 following
		insertion of DDD pacemaker by Dr. Hyde. Upper
		rate limit of 125 bpm and lower rate limit
		of 60 bpm. See attached rhythm strip. No
		arrhythmias noted on monitor. AP 71, BP 128/74,
		RR 18, oral T 97.4° F. Pt. alert and oriented
		to time, place, and person. Skin warm and dry,
		peripheral pulses strong. Lungs clear, normal
		heart sounds. Dressing over R subclavian
		insertion site dry and intact. No c/o discomfort.
		Saline lock in R forearm. Told pt. to report
		any weakness, palpitations, chest pain, dyspnea,
		or prolonged hiccups. ———— Tracy Spencer, RN

Pacemaker (transcutaneous) initiation

- A temporary pacemaker is usually inserted in an emergency; however, in a life-threatening situation, when time is critical, a transcutaneous pacemaker is the best choice.
- This device sends an electrical impulse from the pulse generator to the patient's heart by way of two electrodes, which are placed on the front and back of the patient's chest.
- Transcutaneous pacing is quick and effective, but it's used only until a doctor can establish transvenous pacing.

The write stuff

- Chart the date and time of the procedure.
- Record the reason for transcutaneous pacing and the location of the electrodes.
- Chart the pacemaker settings.
- Note the patient's response to the procedure along with any complications and interventions performed.
- Include rhythm strips from:
  - before and after pacemaker insertion
  - whenever settings are changed
  - when the patient is treated for a complication caused by the pacemaker.
- Record the patient's response to temporary pacing and note changes in his condition.
- Record patient teaching, emotional support, and comfort measures provided.
- If transvenous pacing is ultimately established, document its initiation.

02/15/06	1420	At 1402, pt.'s vitals were AP 32, BP 84/50,
		RR 16. Pt. was arousable with verbal and physical
		stimulation but speech was incomprehensible.
		Skin pale and clammy; peripheral pulses weak.
		Monitor showed bradycardia. Transcutaneous
		pacing initiated at 1408 until transvenous
		pacing can be initiated. Posterior pacing
		electrode placed on ℚ back, below scapulae and
		to the ℚ of the spine. Anterior electrode
		placed on ℚ anterior chest over V₂ to V₅.
		Output set at 40 mA, rate at 60. AP 60,
		BP 94/60, RR 18. Pt. alert and oriented; no c/o
		chest pain, dyspnea, or dizziness. Peripheral
		pulses strong; skin warm and dry. Explained to
		pt. that he may feel a thumping or twitching
		sensation during pacing and to let nurse know
		if discomfort is intolerable so that meds can
		be given. Pt. states he can feel twitching and
		doesn't feel the need for meds at this time.
		———————— Sally Meadows, RN

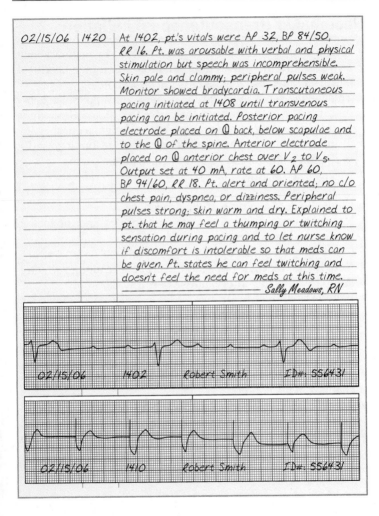

02/15/06   1402   Robert Smith   ID#: 556431

02/15/06   1410   Robert Smith   ID#: 556431

Pacemaker (transvenous) insertion

- A transvenous pacemaker is usually inserted in an emergency by threading an electrode catheter through a vein, such as the brachial, femoral, subclavian, or jugular vein, into the patient's right atrium, right ventricle, or both.
- The electrodes are attached to an external battery-powered pulse generator.

The write stuff

- Record:
  - name of the doctor who inserted the pacemaker
  - date and time the pacemaker was inserted
  - reason for pacing
  - location of the insertion site.
- Document the pacemaker settings.
- Document the patient's level of consciousness and results of your cardiopulmonary assessment, including vital signs.
- Note the patient's response to the procedure as well as any complications and interventions performed.
- Include a rhythm strip in your note.
- Document your assessment of the insertion site.
- Include neurovascular assessment findings of the involved limb, if appropriate.
- Record patient teaching and support given.

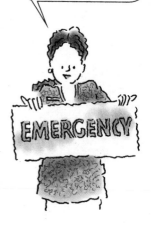

A transvenous pacemaker is usually inserted in an emergency.

02/25/06	1115	Transvenous pacemaker inserted through ®
		subclavian vein by Dr. Peres at 1105 for
		unstable bradycardia. Rate 70, mA 2, full
		demand. 100% ventricular paced rhythm noted
		on monitor. See rhythm strip below. Pt. alert
		and oriented to time, place, and person. Skin
		pale, cool, and dry. Lungs clear, no SOB, normal
		heart sounds, weak dorsalis pedis pulses, and
		no pedal edema bilaterally. AP 70, BP 98/58,
		RR 22, oral T 97.0° F. Radial pulses strong,
		hands warm, no numbness or tingling; pt. is
		able to feel light touch in both hands.
		Insertion site without redness, swelling,
		bleeding, or bruising. Covered with transparent
		semipermeable dressing. Pt. instructed not to
		touch pulse generator and to call the nurse if
		he experiences any light-headedness or
		dizziness. Pt. reports only mild discomfort at
		insertion site but doesn't want any pain med.
		at this time. Pt. resting in bed, chatting with
		wife. ———————— Nicole Stokes, RN

2/25/06   1115   Warrick Braun   ID# 975321

Pacemaker malfunction

- Occasionally, a pacemaker fails to function properly.
- To determine whether your patient's pacemaker is malfunctioning, you'll need to know its mode of function and its settings.
- If a malfunction occurs:
  - notify the practitioner immediately
  - obtain a 12-lead electrocardiogram (ECG)
  - call for a stat chest X-ray, if ordered
  - begin continuous ECG monitoring
  - prepare for temporary pacing.

The write stuff

- Record the date and time of the malfunction.
- Record your patient's signs and symptoms of malfunction, such as dizziness, syncope, irregular pulse, pale skin, dyspnea, chest pain, hypotension, heart rate below the pacemaker's set rate, palpitations, hiccups, and chest or abdominal muscle twitching.
- Place a cardiac rhythm strip in the chart, if possible.
- Note:
  - name of the practitioner notified
  - time of notification
  - orders received (such as obtaining a stat ECG, placing a magnet over a permanent pacemaker, and preparing for temporary pacing).
- Chart your troubleshooting actions, such as:
  - repositioning the patient
  - checking connections and battery settings.
- Document the results of interventions and the patient's response.
- Record patient education and emotional support provided.

07/30/06	1135	Pt. c/o feeling light-headed at 1100. P 54 and
		irregular, BP 92/58, RR 20, oral T 97.4° F.
		Skin pale, lungs clear, normal heart sounds,
		peripheral pulses palpable, no c/o chest pain
		or dyspnea. Pt. has VVI pacemaker set at a
		rate of 68. Pt. attached to portable cardiac
		monitor; rhythm shows intermittent failure to
		pace. Rhythm strip attached below. Notified
		Dr. Steiger at 1105 and dr. came to see pt.
		12-lead ECG confirmed failure to pace. Stat
		CXR done at 1115. Results show lead fracture.
		Dr. Steiger explained to pt. the need to replace
		pacemaker lead. Pt. verbalized understanding
		of procedure and has signed consent form. Dr.
		Steiger calling OR to arrange lead replace-
		ment. Reinforced to pt. that he was being
		monitored closely until he leaves for the OR.
		———————————— Julie Chan, RN

7/30/06	1135	Paul Trudeau	I.D.#: 135789

Pain management

- Your primary goal when caring for a patient with pain is to assess and implement interventions to manage the pain.
- Tools such as a pain flow sheet, visual analog scale, or a graphic rating scale can be used to assess and document pain.
- Interventions to manage pain include:
  - administering analgesics
  - providing emotional support and comfort measures
  - offering alternative therapies to the patient.
- Patients with severe pain may require an opioid analgesic.
- Invasive measures, such as epidural or patient-controlled analgesia, may be required.

The write stuff

- Record the date and time of your entry.
- Describe the location of the pain.
- Record whether the pain interferes with sleep or activities of daily living.
- Describe the pain, using the patient's own words.
- Document how long the pain lasts and how often it occurs.
- Record the patient's ranking of his pain using a pain rating scale.
- Note associated findings, such as grimacing, guarding, pallor, blood pressure changes, dilated pupils, skeletal muscle tension, dyspnea, tachycardia or bradycardia, diaphoresis, nausea, and vomiting.
- Record measures that relieve or heighten the pain.
- Document interventions to alleviate pain and the patient's responses.
- Record patient teaching and emotional support provided.

Assessing and documenting pain

Several tools are available to document pain assessment.

Pain flow sheet
A flow sheet provides a standard for reevaluating a patient's pain at regular intervals.

PAIN FLOW SHEET

Patient name: _Sam Stephens_   Medical record #: _234567_

Date and time	Pain rating (0 to 10)	Patient behaviors	Vital signs	Pain rating after intervention	Comments
01/16/06 0800	7	Wincing, holding head	186/88 98–22	5	Dilaudid 2 mg I.M. given
01/16/06 1200	3	Relaxing, reading	160/80 84–18	2	Tylox † P.O. given

Visual analog pain scale
In a visual analog pain scale, the patient marks a linear scale containing words or numbers that correspond to his perceived degree of pain. Verbal anchors describe the pain's intensity; for example, "no pain" begins the scale and "pain as bad as it could be" ends it. Ask the patient to mark the point on the continuum that best describes his pain.

VISUAL ANALOG SCALE

No pain ————————————— X ————————————— Pain as bad as it could be

Graphic rating scale
Other rating scales have words that represent pain intensity. Use one of these scales as you would the visual analog scale. Have the patient mark the spot on the continuum.

GRAPHIC RATING SCALE

No pain —— Mild —— Moderate X —— Severe —— Pain as bad as it could be

03/19/06	1600	Pt. admitted at 1545 with diagnosis of
		pancreatic cancer and severe pain in LLQ. Pt.
		states, "It feels like my insides are on fire."
		Pt. rates pain as 6 on a scale of 0 to 10, w/
		10 being the worst pain imaginable. States pain
		keeps him from sleeping and eating. States he's
		been taking Percocet 2 tabs q4hr at home, but
		it's no longer providing relief. Pt. alert and
		oriented to time, place, and person. Curled in
		bed on Ⓛ side, with arms wrapped around
		abdomen and softly moaning. Skin pale and
		diaphoretic, pupils dilated. Dr. Martin notified
		of assessment findings at 1550. Dilaudid 2 mg
		ordered and given I.V. P 92, BP 110/64, RR
		22, oral T 99.0° F. Pt. resting at present, no
		longer moaning or curled in a ball. Explained
		pain medication schedule to pt. and reassured
		him that staff will work with him to find
		medications and schedule that reduce his pain
		to a tolerable level. —————— Kate Stout, RN

Patient-controlled analgesia

- A patient-controlled analgesia (PCA) infusion pump allows patients to self-administer boluses of an opioid analgesic I.V. and, sometimes, subcutaneously or epidurally, within limits prescribed by the practitioner.
- To avoid overmedication, an adjustable lockout interval inhibits premature delivery of additional boluses.
- PCA increases the patient's sense of control, reduces anxiety, reduces drug use over the postoperative course, and gives enhanced pain control.
- Indicated for patients who need acute pain control, PCA therapy is typically given to postoperative patients, trauma patients, terminal cancer patients, and other patients with acute pain.

The write stuff

- Record the date and time of your entry; typically, a PCA flow sheet is used.
- Document:
  - name of the opioid used
  - lockout interval
  - maintenance dose
  - amount the patient receives when he activates the device
  - amount of opioid used during your shift.
- Record the patient's assessment of pain relief.
- Include any patient teaching you perform.
- Document your patient's vital signs and level of consciousness, according to policy.
- Record your observations of the insertion site.

Form fitting

PCA flow sheet

A patient-controlled analgesia (PCA) flow sheet documents a patient's self-administration of opioid analgesics. A sample PCA flow sheet is shown below.

Patient name: _Steve Hyde_

Medical record #: _1234567_   Date: _03/22/06_

Medication (Circle one):
Meperidine 300 mg in 30 ml (10 mg/1 ml)   ⟨ Morphine 30 mg in 30 ml (1 mg/ml) ⟩

	7 – 3 shift			
Time (enter in box)	1200	1400		
New cartridge inserted	OR			
PCA settings: lockout interval 7 (minutes)		7		
Dose volume / (ml/dose)				
Four-hour limit: 30 mg				
Continuous settings / (mg/hr)				
Respiratory rate	18	20		
Blood pressure	150/70	130/62		
Sedation rating:				
1. Wide awake	1	2		
2. Drowsy				
3. Dozing, intermittent				
4. Mostly sleeping				
5. Only awakens when stimulated				
Analgesia rts (0 – 10):				
Minimal pain – 1				
Maximum pain – 10	7	8		
Additional doses given (optional doses)	3 ml/OR			
Total ml delivered (total from ampule)	3	6		
ml remaining	27	24		

RN signature (7 – 3 shift) _Brenda Green, RN_   Date _03/22/06_

Patient request to see medical records

- According to the Health Insurance Portability and Accountability Act (HIPAA) of 1996, the patient has the right to view and obtain copies of his medical records.
- Many states have since enacted laws allowing patients access to such records, and health care providers are required to honor such requests.
- When a patient requests to see his medical record, assess why he wants to see it, such as curiosity or concerns about his care.
- Follow facility policy for a patient viewing his own medical record, such as notifying the nursing supervisor, practitioner, legal counsel, and risk manager.
- Explain the procedure for accessing medical records, and give the patient the appropriate forms.
- Use your facility's form or have the patient draft a written request to see his medical record, according to your facility's policy.
- Tell the patient when you expect the records to be available.
- When the medical record is available, properly identify the patient and remain with him while he reads the record.
- Explain that he has the right to request that incorrect information be changed or that missing information be added.
- If the practitioner or health care facility believes that the medical record is correct, the patient can note his disagreement in the medical record.
- Observe how the patient responds while he reads.
- Offer to answer any questions he may have and that the doctor will also answer questions.
- Help the patient interpret abbreviations and jargon used in medical charting.

The write stuff

- Chart the parts of the medical record that the patient requested and whether copies were given to the patient.
- Record the names of the nursing supervisor, risk manager, legal counsel, and practitioner who were notified of the patient's request.
- Record:
  - date and time that the patient reviewed his record
  - name of the person who stayed with the patient while he read it.
- Document the patient's response to reading his record and whether he had questions or concerns.

06/03/06	1400	Pt. stated, "I want to look at my chart." Pt.
		informed that he needed to make request in
		writing. Appropriate forms given to pt. for
		requesting medical records. Pt. complied and
		request sent to medical records. When asked
		why he wanted to see his medical record, pt.
		stated, "I just want to be sure the doctors
		haven't been hiding anything from me."
		Notified Bruce Greenwood, RN, nursing
		supervisor; Loretta Reilly, RN, risk manager;
		and Dr. Felbin of pt.'s request t 1330.
		Identity confirmed by checking ID band
		against chart name and medical record
		number. Dr. Felbin and I were in attendance
		while pt. read record. Pt. asked questions
		regarding terms and abbreviations. Pt.
		appeared calm and relaxed after reading his
		medical record. ———— Henry Williams, R.N

Patient's belongings at admission

- Upon admission, encourage patients to send home their money, jewelry, and other valuable belongings.
- If a patient refuses to do so, make a list of his possessions in your admission note or on an appropriate form and store them according to your facility's policy.
- Place valuable items in an envelope and other personal belongings in approved containers; then label them with the patient's identification number. Give the envelope to security to hold until the patient is discharged, according to your facility's policy.
- Never use garbage containers, laundry bags, or other unauthorized receptacles for valuables because they could be discarded accidentally.

The write stuff

- Make a list of the patient's valuables, with a description of each, to file in the patient's chart; if available, use the appropriate form from your facility.
- Ask the patient (or a responsible family member) to sign or witness the list that you compile so that you both understand the items for which you're responsible.

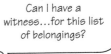

Can I have a witness...for this list of belongings?

- Use objective language to describe each item.
  - Note color, approximate size, style, type, and serial number or other distinguishing features.

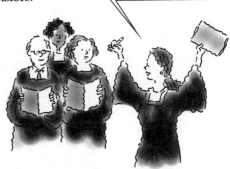

- Don't assess the item's value or authenticity.
- For example, you might describe a diamond ring as a "clear, round stone set in a yellow metal band."
- Include jewelry, money, dentures, eyeglasses or contact lenses, hearing aids, prostheses, and clothing on the list.
- Document that the valuables were sent to security and by whom.

07/09/06	1500	Pt. admitted to ED with one pair of brown
		glasses, upper and lower dentures, a pink
		bathrobe, a radio, a white button shirt, a blue
		skirt, and brown sandals. Pt. will wear a yellow
		metal ring with a red stone on her fourth ⓛ
		finger. $50.00 in cash placed in an envelope
		and labeled with the patient's identification
		number. Envelope given to security officer
		Harrison George. Pt. transferred to room 318
		with belongings. ———————— Paul Cartney, RN

Patient's belongings missing

- A patient's personal belongings may include clothing, eye-glasses, hearing aids, or electronic devices.
- Upon admission, encourage patients to send belongings home with a family member or to lock valuables in the facility's safe.
  - Document that you told them to do so.
  - If items are missing later, you'll have documentation to support your facility's case.
- When a patient believes an item is missing:
  - Check the list of his belongings made on admission (if your facility requires such a list).
  - Ask family members if they took the item home.
  - Help the patient search his room.
  - If the item can't be found, notify security and the nursing supervisor.
- Depending on your facility's policy, you may have a special form on which to document missing items or you may have to complete an incident report.

The write stuff

- Chart the date and time you learned about the missing item.
- Objectively describe the item.
- Record whether the item was on the list of belongings made upon admission.
- Note that you asked family members if they took the item home.
- Include the last time and place the item was seen.
- Describe how you helped the patient search for the item.
- Document:
  - names of the people that you notified, such as security personnel and the nursing supervisor
  - time of notification
  - actions taken.

07/15/06	0900	At 0815, pt. reported his electric razor missing.
		Item was on belongings list made at admission.
		Pt. called wife at home who said she didn't
		take it home. Pt. last remembers using razor
		before surgery. At 845, Eileen Gallen, RN, who
		was caring for pt. before surgery, was called.
		Preop unit called. Razor found in bathroom
		of pt.'s previous room. Volunteer Tom
		Hasenmeyer will bring pt. his razor. ————
		——————————————— Sandy Kelly, RN

Patient self-glucose testing

- A patient with an established diagnosis of diabetes may prefer to use his own glucose meter to test his daily glucose levels.
- Per policy, your facility will require a practitioner's order stating that the patient may use his own glucose meter.
- If your patient is permitted to use his own Food and Drug Administration–approved glucose meter, you must verify his competency by having him demonstrate the procedure to ensure that he's performing it correctly.

Form fitting

Keeping a record of blood glucose levels

Patients performing self-glucose testing while in your facility must keep a record of their blood glucose levels. The nurse provides a chart listing the times when glucose level should be tested or ordered by the practitioner to be tested. Recommendations for the best time of day to test blood glucose level depend on the patient's medicine, meal times, and glucose control.

Name: *Mike Nichols* Date: *03/06/06 – 03/13/06*

Time to test:	Fasting, before breakfast	1 to 2 hours after breakfast	Before lunch
Target goal ranges*:	90 – 130 mg/dl	< 180 mg/dl	90 – 130 mg/dl
Doctor's recommendation	90 – 110 mg/dl	160 mg/dl	90 – 110 mg/dl
Monday	93	159	95
Tuesday	88	159	98
Wednesday	89	161	103
Thursday			
Friday			
Saturday			
Sunday			

* The target goals are based on recommendations from the American Diabetes Association. Talk with your doctor about what changes to make if your blood glucose levels are not within this range.

- Advise the patient to perform quality control testing on the meter according to the manufacturer's guidelines.
- If the patient is using the meter for the first time, correlate the first glucose result from his meter with a fasting blood glucose level drawn by your facility's laboratory.
- Confirm with the patient how and where to record his blood glucose levels.
- Stress the importance of recording results for blood glucose levels.

1 to 2 hours after lunch	Before dinner	1 to 2 hours after dinner	Bedtime	3 a.m
< 180 mg/dl	90 – 130 mg/dl	< 180 mg/dl		
160 mg/dl	90 – 110 mg/dl	160 mg/dl	100 – 130 mg/dl	70 – 130 mg/dl
147	97	158	118	118
143	101	161	112	112
156				

- Inform the patient of blood glucose levels that should be reported immediately.
- Frequency of testing is determined by the practitioner's orders.

The write stuff

- Document that you verified the:
  - practitioner's order allowing the patient to use his glucose meter
  - patient's ability to use his meter by demonstration.
- Record that you compared the patient's first glucose meter reading with the fasting blood glucose level drawn by your facility's laboratory.
- Record the date and time of self-glucose monitoring.
- Document how often the patient performs quality control tests.
- Record the results of the patient's glucose testing.
- Document patient education provided.

02/15/06	1000	Pt. uses his own glucose meter to monitor glucose levels per order by Dr. Alvie Singer using an Optium glucose meter. Pt. demonstrated his ability to properly use his meter. 0800 fasting blood glucose drawn by lab confirmed with pt.'s glucose meter results. Laboratory 0800 fasting blood glucose level was 93 mg/dl. Pt.'s glucose meter reading was 90 mg/dl. Pt. states he checks the quality controls for the meter every day in the morning and checks his blood glucose every day before meals, 2 hours after meals, and at bedtime and 0300 per dr.'s orders. Pt. verbalized how to record glucose levels and when to notify the nurse of the results. —————————————————— Diane Hall, RN

Patient teaching

- Patient and caregiver teaching are essential for:
  - maintaining the patient's health
  - preventing or detecting early signs of complications
  - promoting self-care and independence.
- Teaching is most effective when:
  - it's specific to the patient's and family's physical, financial, emotional, intellectual, cultural, and social circumstances
  - the patient and family are ready to learn, mentally alert, and free from discomfort and distraction.
- Keep teaching sessions short.
- Reinforce all instructions using verbal explanations, demonstrations, videos, and written materials.
- Evaluate the patient's understanding by asking him to:
  - restate material
  - answer your questions
  - give a return demonstration.
- Documentation of your teaching:
  - lets other health care team members know what the patient has been taught and what materials need to be reinforced
  - serves as a record to back you up if the patient files a lawsuit claiming he was injured because he didn't receive instruction.
- Check your facility's policies regarding when, where, and how to document your teaching.
- Patient-teaching forms vary according to the health care facility and may ask you to document information by filling in blanks, checking boxes, or writing brief narrative notes.

The write stuff

- Record the date and time of your entry.
- Document:
  - your assessment of the patient's learning abilities
  - barriers to learning

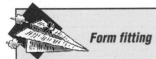

Form fitting

Patient teaching record

PATIENT TEACHING
Instructions for Patients with Diabetes
County Hospital, Waltham, MA

Name: _Bernard Miller_ Admission date: _01/03/06_
Anticipated discharge: _01/08/06_ Diagnosis: _TIA, type 2 DM_

Educational assessment
Comprehension level
Ability to grasp concepts
☑ High
☐ Average
☐ Needs improvement
Comments: _____
_____

Motivational level
☑ Asks questions
☐ Eager to learn
☐ Anxious
☐ Uncooperative
☐ Disinterested
☐ Denies need to learn
Comments: _____
_____

Knowledge and skill levels
Understanding of health condition and how to manage it
☐ High (> 75% working knowledge)
☐ Adequate (50% to 75% working knowledge)
☑ Needs improvement (25% to 50% working knowledge)
☐ Low (< 25% working knowledge)
Comments: _____
_____

Learning barriers
☐ Language (specify: foreign, impairment, laryngectomy, other):
_____
☐ Vision (specify: blind, legally blind, other): ___
_____
☑ Hearing (impaired, deaf) _Need to_ _speak loudly_
☐ Memory
   ☐ Change in long-term memory (specify):
_____
   ☐ Change in short-term memory (specify):
_____
☐ Other (specify):
_____
☐ No learning barriers noted
Instructor's initials: _CW_

Anticipated outcomes
Patient will be prepared to perform self-care at the following level:
☑ High (total self-care)
☐ Moderate (self-care with minor assistance)
☐ Minimal (self-care with more than 50% assistance)

Patient teaching record *(continued)*

Key

P = Patient taught
F = Caregiver or family taught
R = Reinforced

N/A = Not applicable
A = Asked questions
B = Nonattentive, poor concentration

C = Expressed denial, resistance
D = Verbalized recall
E = Demonstrated ability

Date	01/04/06	01/05/06	01/05/06	01/05/06
Time	1900	0800	1330	1830
Assessed educational needs				
Assessment of patient's (or caregiver's) current knowledge of disease (include medical, family, and social histories)	A/CW			
Assessment of learner's reaction to diagnosis (verbal and nonverbal responses)	A/CW			
General diabetic education goals The patient (or caregiver) will:				
• define diabetes mellitus.	P/A/CW	R/EG	D/ME	
• state hormone produced in the pancreas.	P/A/CW	R/EG	D/ME	
• identify three signs and symptoms of diabetes.	P/CW	R/EG	D/ME	
• discuss risk factors associated with diabetes.	P/CW	R/EG	D/ME	
• differentiate between type 1 and type 2 diabetes.	P/A/CW	R/EG	D/ME	
Survival skill goals The patient (or caregiver) will:				
• identify the name, purpose, dose, and time of administration of medication ordered.		P/EG	R/ME	D/LT
• properly administer insulin.	N/A			
– draw up insulin properly.	N/A			
– discuss and demonstrate site selection and rotation.	N/A			
– demonstrate proper injection technique with needle angled appropriately.	N/A			
– explain correct way to store insulin.	N/A			
– demonstrate correct disposal of syringes.	N/A			

(continued)

Patient teaching record *(continued)*

Key
P = Patient taught
F = Caregiver or family taught
R = Reinforced

N/A = Not applicable
A = Asked questions
B = Nonattentive, poor concentration

C = Expressed denial, resistance
D = Verbalized recall
E = Demonstrated ability

Date	01/04/06	01/05/06	01/05/06	01/05/06
Time	1900	0800	1330	1830
Survival skill goals *(continued)*				
• distinguish among types of insulin.	N/A			
– species (pork or recombinant DNA)	N/A			
– regular	N/A			
– NPH/Ultralente (longer acting)	N/A			
• properly administer mixed insulins.	N/A			
– demonstrate injecting air into vials.	N/A			
– draw up mixed insulin properly (regular before NPH).	N/A			
• demonstrate knowledge of oral antidiabetic agents.				
– identify name of medication, dose, and time of administration.		P/EG	A/ME	
– identify purpose of medication.		P/EG	A/ME	
– state possible adverse effects.		P/EG	A/ME	
• list signs and symptoms, causes, implications, and treatments of hyperglycemia and hypoglycemia.		P/EG	A/ME	
• monitor blood glucose levels satisfactorily.				
– demonstrate proper use of blood glucose monitoring device.				P/LT
– perform fingerstick.				P/LT
– obtain accurate blood glucose reading.				P/LT

Patient teaching record (continued)

Key

P = Patient taught
F = Caregiver or family taught
R = Reinforced

N/A = Not applicable
A = Asked questions
B = Nonattentive, poor concentration

C = Expressed denial, resistance
D = Verbalized recall
E = Demonstrated ability

Date	01/04/06	01/05/06	01/05/06	01/05/06
Time	1900	0800	1330	1830
Healthful living goals The patient (or caregiver) will:				
• consult with the nutritionist about meal planning.			P/ME	R/LT
• follow the diet recommended by the American Diabetes Association.			P/ME	R/LT
• state importance of adhering to diet.			P/ME	R/LT
• give verbal feedback on 1-day meal plan.			P/ME	R/LT
• state the effects of stress, illness, and exercise on blood glucose levels.			P/ME	R/LT
• state when to test urine for ketones and how to address results.			P/ME	R/LT
• identify self-care measures for periods when illness occurs.			P/ME	R/LT
• list precautions to take while exercising.			P/ME	R/LT
• explain what steps to take when patient doesn't want to eat or drink on proper schedule.			P/ME	R/LT
• agree to wear medical identification (for example, a Medic Alert bracelet).			P/ME	R/LT
Safety goals The patient (or caregiver) will:				
• state the possible complications of diabetes.	P/CW	R/EG		D/LT
• explain the importance of careful, regular skin care.	P/CW	R/EG		D/LT

(continued)

Patient teaching record (continued)

Key
P = Patient taught
F = Caregiver or family taught
R = Reinforced

N/A = Not applicable
A = Asked questions
B = Nonattentive, poor concentration

C = Expressed denial, resistance
D = Verbalized recall
E = Demonstrated ability

Date	01/04/06	01/05/06	01/05/06	01/05/06
Time	1900	0800	1330	1830
Safety goals (continued)				
• demonstrate healthful foot care.	P/CW	R/EG		D/LT
• discuss the importance of regular eye care and examinations.	P/CW	R/EG		D/LT
• state the importance of oral hygiene	P/CW	R/EG		D/LT
Individual goals				

Initial	Signature				
CW	Carol Witt, RN, BSN				
EG	Ellie Grimes, RN, MSN				
ME	Marianne Evans, RN				
LT	Lynn Tata, RN, BSN				

- goals to be met
- equipment or supplies used
- specific content taught
- response to teaching
- skills to be acquired by the time of discharge.
- Chart how you evaluated the patient's learning, such as by return demonstration or verbalization of understanding.
- Before discharge, document:
  - patient's remaining learning needs
  - whether you provided him with printed material or other patient-teaching aids.

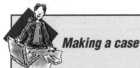 *Making a case*

Documenting what you teach

Always document what you teach the patient and his family and their understanding of what you taught. Such documentation can be helpful in court.

Case in point

The court in *Kyslinger v. United States* (1975) addressed the nurse's liability for patient teaching. In this case, a veterans' administration (VA) hospital sent a hemodialysis patient home with an artificial kidney. He eventually died (apparently while on the hemodialysis machine) and his wife sued, alleging that the hospital and its staff failed to teach either her or her late husband how to properly use and maintain a home hemodialysis unit.

Judgment day

After examining the evidence, the court ruled against the patient's wife, as follows: "During those 10 months that plaintiff's decedent underwent biweekly hemodialysis treatment on the unit (at the VA hospital), both plaintiff and decedent were instructed as to the operation, maintenance, and supervision of said treatment. The Court can find no basis to conclude that the plaintiff or plaintiff's decedent were not properly informed on the use of the hemodialysis unit."

Patient transfer to alternate care facility

- As much as 25% of older adults need long-term care assistance.
- Various levels of care are offered at alternate care facilities:
  - Assisted living facilities and adult homes provide meals, sheltered living, and some medical monitoring for patients who don't need continuous medical attention.
  - Intermediate care facilities provide custodial care for individuals who are unable to care for themselves due to mental or physical infirmities, including physical, social, and recreational activities and, sometimes, rehabilitation.
  - Skilled nursing facilities provide medical supervision, rehabilitation services, and 24-hour nursing care by registered nurses, licensed practical nurses, and nurses' aides for patients who have the potential to regain function.
- Patients are discharged from the hospital and transferred to an appropriate facility for one of the levels of care described.
- A transfer form is typically completed for discharge to intermediate care and skilled nursing facilities.
- When a patient is transferred, copies of sections of the medical record may be sent with the patient. Check your facility's policy.

The write stuff

- Record:
  - date and time of the discharge
  - practitioner's name
  - that discharge orders were written
  - long-term care facility's name
  - name of the nurse who received your verbal report.
- Note if discharge instructions were discussed with the patient and a copy given to him.

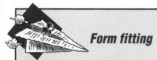

Form fitting

Patient transfer form

PATIENT TRANSFER FORM			
Patient's Name (Last, First, M.I.) *Davis, Gladys*		Sex: ☐ M ☑ F	Date of birth: *10/11/43*
Patient's address: *139 Hillside Drive, Springville, PA*			
Date of this transfer: *6/20/06*		Facility name and address transferring to: *The Manor, Hartwick, PA*	
Physician in charge at time of transfer: *Dr. J. Cannon*			Physician phone number: *867-555-5309*

Diagnosis at time of transfer
Primary: *Right-sided heart failure*
Secondary: *Pulmonary embolism, heart failure, angina*

Vital signs at time of transfer:				Transfer orders – Medications or respiratory therapy
T	P	R	BP	*Oxygen 2 to 3 L by nasal prongs as needed for*
98	76	22	119/56	*oxygen saturation less than 93%*

Diet: *Low salt, fluid restrictions*

Teaching: CXR and 12-lead ECG for SOB or angina
Daily weights
Monitor I & O
Medications:
  Digoxin 0.125 mg PO daily

Allergies: *Sulfa, PCN*

  Furosemide 40 mg PO daily
  Coumadin 4 mg PO daily – call Dr. Cannon with
    weekly INR for dosing
  Captopril 25 mg PO bid

Past medical history:
Peripheral neuropathy, atrial fibrillation, HTN, cholecystectomy

  Metoprolol long acting 25 mg PO daily
  Enalapril 2.5 mg PO daily
  Acetaminophen 650 mg PO PRN
Follow-up appointments: *6/28 at 2:15 pm*
  with Dr. Cannon
Advance directives: *Living will and health care*
  proxy with chart

Pneumococcal vaccine
Date: *6/15/06*

Follow-up diagnostics: *CXR, ECG 6/27 call results to*
Dr. Cannon
Follow-up labs: Is patient on warfarin? ☐ N ☑ Y
  If yes, next INR: *6/27*

Influenza vaccine
Date: *6/15/06*

BMP, CBC, BNP 6/27 call results to Dr. Cannon
Eval and treatment: ☑ PT ☑ OT ☐ Speech

Signature of physician: *J. Cannon, MD* Print Name: *J. Cannon* Date: *6/20/06*

(continued)

Patient transfer form *(continued)*

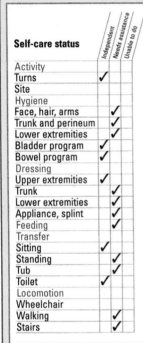

Self-care status	Independent	Needs assistance	Unable to do
Activity			
Turns	✓		
Site			
Hygiene			
Face, hair, arms		✓	
Trunk and perineum		✓	
Lower extremities		✓	
Bladder program	✓		
Bowel program	✓		
Dressing			
Upper extremities	✓		
Trunk		✓	
Lower extremities		✓	
Appliance, splint		✓	
Feeding		✓	
Transfer			
Sitting	✓		
Standing		✓	
Tub		✓	
Toilet	✓		
Locomotion			
Wheelchair			
Walking		✓	
Stairs		✓	

Mental status: *Oriented x 3, forgetful at times*

Communication ability: *Speech clear, slightly hard of hearing*

Disabilities: *None*

Incontinence: *None*

Prosthesis/appliance: *Bilateral leg braces with shoes and walker*

Dentures: *Upper*

Other equipment: *Ambulation with assistance and use of walker*

Clinical notes – additional pertinent information (Explain necessary details for care, diagnosis, medications, treatments, prognosis, teaching, habits, preferences, etc. Therapists and social workers add signature and title to notes.)

Mrs. Davis was admitted to Valley View Hospital on 6/6/06 for acute SOB and subsequent findings of a PE. Pt. received TPA with resolution of symptoms and resulting right-sided heart failure with ejection fraction of 20%. Pt. is recovering well with no complications. Requires much assistance due to weakness and will need medication adjustments for chronic heart failure, and education for patient and family in preparation to discharge home in 4 weeks. Plan daily activities to avoid SOB and keep patients legs elevated when OOB. –

Current labs:
Hg — 12.8 g/dL
BUN — 25 mg/dL
Creat — 1.5 mg/dL
K — 4.2 mEg/L
BNP — 480 pg/mL

Activity tolerance: *SOB with ADLs*

Potential for rehabilitation: *Fair*

Activity and exercises: *Follow PT and OT evaluations. Walk 6 times/day*

Wound care treatment:

Skin integrity (Document any red areas or disruption of skin integrity at time of transfer)

Pressure ulcers: *Reddened heels*

- Chart if belongings were transferred with the patient or that the patient signed a personal belongings form acknowledging that he has all his belongings. Document that the form was placed in the medical record.
- Describe the condition of your patient at discharge, including:
  - vital signs
  - descriptions of wounds
  - tubes or other equipment that's still in place.
- Record the time of discharge from the hospital and transfer to the alternate care facility as well as who accompanied the patient, the mode of transportation, and the name of the person at the alternate care facility who will be receiving him.
- Indicate whether the medical record was copied and sent with the patient.
- Document whether a transfer form was completed and whether a copy was sent to the receiving facility.
- Include the following information, per policy, on the transfer form:
  - demographic patient information
  - financial information
  - receiving facility information
  - medical information, including diagnoses, surgeries, allergies, laboratory test values, and advance directives
  - family contacts
  - services needed, such as physical, occupational, or speech therapy; dialysis; or wound management

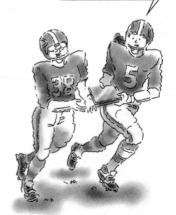

Use proper charting to tell those on the receiving end of a transfer about a patient's condition.

- practitioner's information and orders
- medication information that includes a list of all of the medications the patient is receiving, including last dose given
- assessment of body systems
- ability to perform activities of daily living.

| 05/11/06 | 1300 | Pt. transferred to Orleans Skilled Nursing Facility at 1230. Pt. transported by stretcher via Metro ambulance. Personal belongings list completed and placed in chart. Copy placed with belongings sent with pt. Pt. unable to sign belongings form. Transfer orders written by Dr. DeStat. Verbal report given to Claudia Peters, RN, who will be receiving pt. Transfer forms completed, copy sent with pt. Copy of medical records also sent with pt. At the time of discharge, pt. alert and oriented to person but not to place, date, and time. P 72, BP 128/70, RR 18, oral T 98.2° F. Lungs clear with diminished breath sounds at bases, normal heart sounds, positive bowel sounds in all 4 quadrants, incontinent of bladder and bowels. Skin warm, dry, pedal pulses palpable, no edema. Has stage 2 ulcer on coccyx, 2 cm X 2 cm and approximately 2 mm deep, red granulation tissue at base, transparent dressing covering wound. See referral form for treatments and medication reconciliation list for current medications. ——— Annie Rice, RN |

Patient transfer to specialty unit

- Specialty units provide continuous and intensive monitoring and care to patients.
- Specialty units include perioperative units, labor and delivery units, burn units, and the many types of intensive care units.
- Specialty units rely on close and continuous assessment by registered nurses as well as technological monitoring.
- Medication administration is complex and frequent; measurements are performed hourly or more frequently.
- Some facilities may use a transfer form to record transfer information.

The write stuff

- Record the date and time of the transfer and the name of the unit receiving the patient.
- Document that you received transfer orders.
- Describe the patient's condition at the time of transfer, including:
  - vital signs
  - descriptions of incisions and wounds
  - locations of tubes or medical devices still in place.
- Report significant events that occurred during the hospital stay.
- Note whether the patient has advance directives.
- Document special factors, such as allergies, special diet, sensory deficits, and language or cultural issues.
- List the patient's current medications, treatments, and teaching needs.
- Note which goals were and weren't met.
- Chart that you gave a report to the receiving unit; include the name of the nurse who received the report.
- Note how the patient was transported to the specialty unit and who accompanied him.

- Include patient teaching given that related to the transfer (such as explaining to the patient why he's being transferred).

05/24/06	1430	Pt. is 63 y.o. white English-speaking female, with
		early Alzheimer's disease, being transferred
		from medical unit to MICU by stretcher
		accompanied by her daughter Mary Golden and
		medical resident Brian Wilson. Report given to
		Natalie Brown, RN. Advance directives in chart.
		Pt. unresponsive to verbal stimuli, opens eyes
		to painful stimuli. Prior to this episode,
		daughter reports pt. was alert and oriented
		to person but not always to place and time.
		Daughter states that pt.'s forgetfulness and
		confusion have recently gotten worse. Pt. was
		found alone in her apartment 2 days ago. No
		food eaten or dishes used since last groceries
		purchased for pt. 2 days ago. Pt. is dehydrated
		despite 2000 ml over last 24 hr. Currently
		NPO. I.V. infusion with 18G catheter in ®
		antecubital vein with 0.45% NSS at 75 ml/hr.
		AP 124 irregular, BP 84/palp, RR 28, rectal
		T 100.0° F, weight 78 lb., height 64". Allergies
		to molds, pollen, and mildew. Lungs clear,
		normal heart sounds. Skin intact, pale, cool,
		poor skin turgor. Radial pulses weak, pedal
		pulses not palpable. Foley catheter in place
		draining approx. 30 ml/hr. Orders written by
		Dr. Jordan to transfer patient to special care
		unit. Medical record, MAR, and nursing Kardex
		transferred with pt. Pt's daughter understands
		reason for transfer to MICU. ————————
		——————————— Sarah Harmer, RN

Peripherally inserted central catheter insertion

- A peripherally inserted central catheter (PICC) allows for safe, reliable access for drug administration and blood sampling.
- For a patient who needs central venous (CV) therapy for 1 to 6 months or requires repeated venous access, a PICC may be the best option.
- PICCs are:
  - made of silicone or polyurethane
  - soft and flexible with increased biocompatibility
  - available in single and double lumens
  - easier to insert than other CV devices
  - safe, reliable modes of access for drug administration and blood sampling.
- The practitioner may order a PICC:
  - to avoid complications of a CV line
  - if the patient has suffered trauma or burns resulting in chest injury
  - if he has respiratory compromise due to chronic obstructive pulmonary disease, a mediastinal mass, cystic fibrosis, or pneumothorax.
- PICCs are being used increasingly for patients receiving home care infusions.
- Infusions commonly given by PICC include total parenteral nutrition, chemotherapy, antibiotics, opioids, and analgesics.
- Some state nurse practice acts permit nurses to insert PICC lines; those that do require that nurses receive certification after mandatory course work and successful supervised practice.

The write stuff

- Record the date and time of insertion.
- Document that the procedure has been explained to the patient, all questions have been answered, and informed consent has been obtained.

- Document the entire procedure, including problems with catheter placement.
- Chart the size, length, and type of catheter as well as the insertion site.
- Record flush solutions.
- Describe the dressing applied.
- Document that a chest X-ray verified tip placement before initial use.
- Record the patient's tolerance of the procedure.
- Document any patient education given.

| 06/30/06 | 1200 | PICC insertion procedure explained to pt. and her husband John. Informed consent obtained. After asking many questions about PICC care, pt. and husband verbalized understanding of the procedure. Antecubital-shoulder-sternal notch measurement 20¼". Using sterile technique, PICC cut to 23¼". Extension tubing and catheter flushed w/NSS. Ⓛ basilic vein site prepared with chlorhexidine. With pt. in supine position and Ⓛ arm at 90-degree angle, catheter introducer inserted into vein at 10-degree angle; blood return noted. Catheter introduced and advanced to shoulder. Instructed pt. to turn head Ⓛ and place chin on chest. Catheter then advanced until only 4" remained. Introducer sheath removed, and catheter advanced until completely inserted. Catheter flushed with NSS followed by heparin. See MAR. 2" X 2" gauze pad placed over site, covered by sterile transparent semipermeable dressing. CXR done at 1150 to check tip placement; results pending. Following procedure, pt. sitting up in bed talking with husband. No c/o pain, except for "minor" discomfort at insertion site. ———————— *Anita Worthington, RN* |

Peripherally inserted central catheter site care

- Proper site care and dressing changes are vital to preventing infection.
- After the initial insertion of a peripherally inserted central catheter (PICC), a new sterile, transparent, semipermeable dressing is applied.
- Thereafter, the dressing should be changed:
  - every 3 to 7 days, according to your facility's policy
  - as needed
  - if it becomes wet or soiled or it loses integrity.
- Assess the catheter insertion site through the transparent semipermeable dressing every 24 hours, or per your facility's policy.
- Look at the catheter and cannula pathway, and check for bleeding, redness, drainage, and swelling.
- Ask the patient if he has pain at the site.

The write stuff

- Record the date and time of site care.
- Note that you have explained the procedure to the patient and answered his questions.
- Describe the condition of the site, noting any bleeding, redness, drainage, and swelling.
- Document pain or discomfort reported by the patient and your interventions.
- Note:
  - name of the practitioner notified of complications

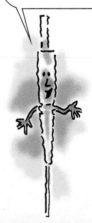

Be "PICC-y" about your PICC site care documentation. Record the condition of the site, including the presence of bleeding, swelling, or drainage.

- time of notification
- orders received
- your interventions
- patient's response to interventions.
• Record how the site was cleaned and the type of dressing applied.
• Document the patient's tolerance of the procedure.
• Document patient teaching you provide.

11/30/06	1100	Explained dressing change and site care for
		PICC to pt. Pt. verbalized understanding.
		Placed pt. in seated position with ⓛ arm at
		45-degree angle from body. Old dressing
		removed, no redness, bleeding, drainage, or
		swelling. No c/o pain at site. Using sterile
		technique, site cleaned with chlorhexidine.
		Sterile, transparent, semipermeable dressing
		applied and tubing secured to edge of
		dressing with tape. Pt. reports no pain or
		tenderness following the dressing change.
		Reminded pt. to report pain or discomfort at
		insertion site or in ⓛ arm to nurse. ————
		———————————————— Lillian Mott, RN

Peritoneal dialysis

- Peritoneal dialysis is indicated for patients with chronic kidney failure who have cardiovascular instability, vascular access problems that prevent hemodialysis, fluid overload, or electrolyte imbalances.
- In this procedure, dialysate—the solution instilled into the peritoneal cavity by a catheter—draws waste products, excess fluid, and electrolytes from the blood across the semipermeable peritoneal membrane.
- After a prescribed period, the dialysate is drained from the peritoneal cavity, removing impurities with it.
- The dialysis procedure is then repeated, using a new dialysate each time until waste removal is complete and fluid, electrolyte, and acid-base balances have been restored.
- Peritoneal dialysis may be performed manually or by using an automatic or semiautomatic cycle machine.

The write stuff

- Record the date and time of dialysis.
- During and after dialysis, monitor and document the patient's response to treatment.
- Record vital signs according to your facility's policy.
- Document:
  - changes in the patient's condition
  - abnormalities in the dialysate
  - name of the practitioner notified
  - time of notification
  - orders received.
- Record the amount of dialysate infused and drained and medications added.
- Keep a record of the effluent's characteristics and the assessed negative or positive fluid balance at the end of each infusion-dwell-drain cycle.
- Chart the patient's weight (immediately after the drain phase) and abdominal girth daily, noting:

- time of day
- variations in the weighing-measuring technique.
- Document physical assessment findings and fluid status daily.
- Keep a record of equipment problems, such as kinked tubing or mechanical malfunction, and your interventions.
- Note:
  - condition of the patient's skin at the dialysis catheter site
  - patient's reports of unusual discomfort or pain
  - interventions performed.
- Complete a peritoneal dialysis flow chart every 24 hours.
- Use the appropriate flow sheets for frequent vital signs and intake and output.

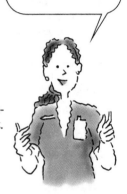

For patients receiving peritoneal dialysis, charting daily weight and abdominal girth measurements is essential.

| 01/15/06 | 0700 | Pt. receiving exchanges q2hr of 1500 ml 4.25 dialysate with 500 units heparin and 2 mEq KCL. Dialysate infused over 15 min. Dwell time 75 min. Drain time 30 min. Drainage clear, pale-yellow fluid. Weight 135 lb, abdominal girth 40" after drain phase. Lungs clear, normal heart sounds, mucous membranes moist, no skin tenting when pinched. VSS (See flow sheets for fluid balance and frequent VS assessments.) No c/o cramping or discomfort. Skin warm, dry at RLQ catheter site, no redness or drainage. Dry split 4" X 4" dressing applied after site cleaned per protocol. —————— Liz Schaeffer, RN |

Peritoneal lavage

- Used as a diagnostic procedure in a patient with blunt abdominal trauma, peritoneal lavage helps detect bleeding in the peritoneal cavity.
- Initially, the doctor inserts a catheter through the abdominal wall into the peritoneal cavity and aspirates the peritoneal fluid with a syringe.
- If the doctor can't see blood in the aspirated fluid, he then infuses a balanced saline solution and siphons the fluid from the cavity.
- The doctor inspects the siphoned fluid for blood and also sends fluid samples to the laboratory for microscopic examination.

The write stuff

- Record the date and time of the procedure.
- Chart teaching done to prepare the patient for the procedure.
- Frequently monitor and document the patient's vital signs and signs and symptoms of shock (for example, tachycardia, hypotension, diaphoresis, or dyspnea).
- Note whether an indwelling urinary catheter or nasogastric (NG) tube was inserted before the procedure.
- Record the size and type of urinary catheter or NG tube used.
- Describe the amount, color, and other characteristics of the urine or NG drainage.
- Keep a record of the catheter site's condition.
- Document:
  – type and size of peritoneal dialysis catheter used
  – type and amount of solution instilled and withdrawn from the peritoneal cavity
  – amount and color of fluid returned.
- Note whether the fluid flowed freely into and out of the abdomen.

- Record which specimens were obtained and sent to the laboratory.
- Note the patient's tolerance of the procedure.
- Document any complications and interventions performed.

01/02/06	1500	NG tube inserted at 1445 via ® nostril and
		connected to low continuous suction, draining
		small amount of greenish colored fluid;
		hematest negative. #16 Fr. Foley catheter
		inserted to straight drainage. Drained 200 ml
		clear amber urine, negative for blood. Dr.
		Gleave inserted #15 peritoneal dialysis
		catheter below umbilicus via trocar. Clear fluid
		withdrawn. 700 ml warm NSS instilled as
		ordered and clamped. Pt. turned from side to
		side. NSS dwell time of 10 min. 650 ml fluid
		returned. NSS drained freely from abdomen.
		Fluid samples sent to lab, as ordered.
		Peritoneal catheter removed and incision
		closed by Dr. Gleave. 4" X 4" gauze pad with
		povidone-iodine ointment applied to site. Pt.
		resting comfortably in semi-Fowler's position.
		No c/o pain or cramping. Breathing
		comfortably. Preprocedure P 92, BP 110/64, RR
		24. Postprocedure P 88, BP 116/66, RR 18. ———
		——————— Joan Keyburn, RN

Pneumonia

- An acute infection of the lung parenchyma, pneumonia commonly impairs gas exchange.
- The prognosis is generally good for people who have normal lungs and adequate host defenses before the onset of pneumonia.
- If your patient has pneumonia, administer antibiotics, as ordered, and provide for good respiratory hygiene.

The write stuff

- Record the date and time of your entry.
- Document your assessment findings, such as coughing, pleuritic chest pain, fever, malaise, abnormal breath sounds, and dullness to percussion over consolidated areas.
- Note:
  - name of the practitioner notified
  - time of notification
  - orders received (such as to obtain a chest X-ray and blood and sputum cultures).
- Record your interventions, such as:
  - administering antibiotics, antipyretics, and oxygen therapy
  - providing a high-calorie diet
  - promoting rest
  - performing chest physiotherapy and postural drainage
  - encouraging incentive spirometry and coughing and deep breathing
  - providing comfort measures and analgesics.
- Document the patient's response to interventions.

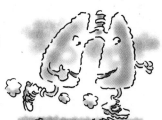

Remember to document that you encouraged your patient to exercise his lungs.

- Use flow sheets to record:
  - frequent assessments
  - vital signs
  - intake and output
  - I.V. therapy
  - laboratory test values.
- Record patient education given.

12/24/06	0900	Pt. has cough productive for large amount of thick yellow sputum. Breath sounds diminished to base of ① lower lung, crackles throughout all lung fields bilaterally. Dullness to percussion and tactile fremitus heard over base of ① lung. Pt. is SOB, using accessory breathing muscles. P 112, BP 152/88, RR 32 and shallow, rectal T 102.4° F. Pulse oximetry 91%. Pt. is shaking and c/o of chills, weakness, and malaise. Normal heart sounds. Skin hot, dry, peripheral pulses palpable, no edema. Pt. alert and oriented to time, place, and person. Notified Dr. Flanders at 0845 of assessment findings. Per dr.'s orders, chest X-ray and blood cultures ordered. Sputum sent for culture and sensitivity. Placed pt. on 2 L humidified O_2 by NC. Pulse oximetry 96%. Explained all procedures to pt. Showed pt. how to perform cough and deep-breathing exercises and encouraged him to perform them q2hr. Pt. able to give proper return demo. —————— *Henry Potter, RN*

Pneumothorax

- Pneumothorax is an accumulation of air in the pleural space, which leads to partial or complete lung collapse.
- A closed pneumothorax:
  - has no associated external wound
  - is commonly caused by the rupture of small blebs in the lung's visceral pleural space.
- An open pneumothorax:
  - develops when air enters the pleural space through an opening in the external chest wall
  - is commonly associated with a stab or gunshot wound.
- With a tension pneumothorax:
  - Intra-thoracic pressure increases.
  - The lung collapses and the mediastinum shifts toward the side opposite the pneumothorax.
  - Venous return decreases and great vessels compress.
  - Cardiac output decreases, creating an emergency situation.
- If you suspect your patient has a pneumothorax, contact the practitioner immediately and anticipate an immediate chest X-ray and insertion of a chest tube.

The write stuff

- Record the date and time of your entry.
- Document assessment findings suggestive of pneumothorax, such as asymmetrical chest wall movement, shortness of breath, decreased oxygen saturation, pain exacerbated by breathing, and tracheal deviation (in tension pneumothorax).
- Document whether a chest X-ray was obtained.
- Note:
  - name of the practitioner notified
  - time of notification
  - orders received.
- Record your interventions, such as:
  - obtaining an immediate chest X-ray
  - administering oxygen

- assisting with insertion of a chest tube or large-bore needle
- managing the chest tube
- encouraging coughing and deep-breathing exercises.
- Document the patient's response to interventions.
- Use flow sheets to record:
  - frequent cardiopulmonary assessments
  - vital signs
  - intake and output
  - I.V. therapy
  - chest X-ray results
  - laboratory values.
- Include patient teaching and emotional care given.

| 07/12/06 | 0200 | Pt. entered ED at 0130 with c/o difficulty breathing and Ⓛ-sided chest pain that worsened with movement; has history of COPD. Breath sounds absent on Ⓛ side, clear breath sounds on Ⓡ. Skin pale, cool. Normal heart sounds; however, PMI is shifted to Ⓡ of midclavicular line. P 128 and weak, BP 112/62, RR 32, axillary T 99.0° F. Pulse oximetry 84% on room air. O₂ applied at 30% via facemask. Dr. Flansberg in to see pt. at 0140 and orders given. Portable CXR done and reveals Ⓛ pneumothorax. Chest tube inserted in Ⓛ chest by Dr. Hall at 0150 and placed to water seal drainage with 20 cm water suction with Pleur-evac. Chest tube sutured to chest wall. Airtight dressing applied. I.V. line inserted in Ⓡ forearm on first attempt using 18G catheter. 500 ml NSS infusing at 30 ml/hr. Pt. states he's breathing easier. No dyspnea noted. P 110 and strong, BP 118/60, RR 24. See flow sheets for documentation of frequent VS, I/O, I.V. therapy, and lab values. ———— John Linnel, RN |

Police custody of patient

- A patient in police custody may be admitted voluntarily for medical or surgical treatment or involuntarily for psychiatric care.
- Follow your facility's policy for caring for a patient in police custody.
- Safety considerations include removal of objects from the patient care area that the patient could use to harm himself or others.
- The accompanying police officer isn't permitted to make decisions regarding the patient's medical care and treatment.
- The patient is afforded the rights of:
  - confidentiality
  - informed consent
  - refusal of treatment
  - review of documents that describe his condition and care.
- All care must be delivered without discrimination.
- A competent patient in police custody has the right to make his own treatment decisions.
- If blood, urine, or other samples are collected:
  - don't leave them unattended
  - follow facility policy for using a chain of custody form, which serves as an uninterrupted log of the whereabouts of the evidence.
- Documentation of care should be equivalent to that provided for any patient, with special attention to documenting the presence of a police officer and visitors.

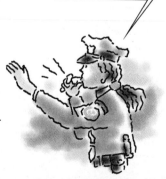

Stop in the name of the law! And document the name and badge number of the officer guarding your patient.

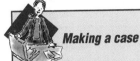

Making a case

When a prisoner refuses treatment

Several courts have stated that individuals have a constitutional right to privacy based on a high regard for human dignity and self-determination. That means any competent adult may refuse medical care, even lifesaving treatments. A suspected criminal may refuse unwarranted bodily invasions. However, an arrested suspect or convicted criminal doesn't have the same right to refuse lifesaving measures.

Case in point
In *Commissioner of Correction v. Myers* (1979), a prisoner with renal failure refused hemodialysis unless he was moved to a minimum-security prison.

Judgment day
The court determined that, although the defendant's imprisonment didn't divest him of his right to privacy or his interest in maintaining his bodily integrity, it did impose limitations on those constitutional rights.

Practical practice
As a practical matter, any time a patient refuses lifesaving treatments, inform your facility's administration. In the case of a suspect or prisoner, notify law enforcement authorities as well.

The write stuff

- Record the name and badge number of the officer guarding your patient.
- Note safety measures taken in preparing the patient care area.
- Document that the patient's rights were protected.
- Note tests and treatments and the patient's responses to them.

- If you turn anything over to the police or administration, record what it is and the name of the person receiving it.
- Record a suspect's statements that are directly related to his care only.
- Document all specific instructions given for follow-up care; this documentation may be critical, especially if the patient claims he was mistreated.
- Note that you gave a copy of the discharge instructions to the patient and the police officer.

08/02/06	0800	Pt. admitted to ED at 0730 with head
		laceration from MVA. Pt. accompanied by San
		Antonio police officer B. Starr, badge #4532.
		Pt. placed in private exam room for privacy
		and safety. Officer in attendance at all times.
		Pt. alert, oriented to time, place, and person.
		Speech clear and coherent. PERRLA. Lungs
		clear, normal heart sounds, all peripheral
		pulses palpable. P 82, BP 138/74, RR 18 and
		unlabored, oral T 97.7° F. Pt. moves all
		extremities on own, no deformities noted. No
		c/o nausea, vomiting, dizziness, diplopia, pain,
		except for sore forehead. Dr. Lawson in to see
		pt at 0740. Cleaned head wound and applied
		sterile 4" X 4" dressing to 2-cm cut on ® side
		of forehead. Orders written for pt. discharge.
		Explained wound care to pt. and police
		officer, s/s to report to doctor. Written
		instructions for wound care and head injury
		given to pt. and police officer. Both pt. and
		police officer verbalized understanding of
		instructions. ———————— Joe Purdy, R.N

Postoperative care

- When your patient recovers sufficiently from the effects of anesthesia, he can be transferred from the postanesthesia care unit (PACU) to his unit for ongoing recovery and care.
- Documentation should reflect frequent assessments and interventions.
- The frequency of assessments depends on:
  - facility's policy
  - practitioner's orders
  - patient's condition.
- Compare your assessments to preoperative and PACU assessments.

The write stuff

- Record the date and time of each entry.
- Note the time the patient returned to your nursing unit.
- Chart your assessment of airway and breathing, including:
  - breath sounds
  - positioning to maintain a patent airway
  - use of oxygen
  - respiratory rate, rhythm, and depth.
- Include the patient's vital signs.
- Document your neurologic assessment, including level of consciousness.
- Note the condition of any wounds, including appearance of:
  - dressing
  - drainage
  - bleeding
  - skin around site.
- Document the presence of drainage tubes and amount, type, color, and consistency of drainage; include the type and amount of suction, if applicable.

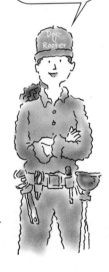

I got a call that some drainage needs documenting.

- Record your cardiovascular assessment, including:
  - heart rate and rhythm
  - peripheral pulses
  - skin color and temperature
  - Homans' sign.
- Record your renal assessment, including:
  - urine output
  - patency of catheter
  - bladder distention.
- Record your GI assessment, including:
  - bowel sounds
  - abdominal distention
  - nausea or vomiting.
- Include a pain assessment, using a 0-to-10 rating scale.
- Document the need for analgesics or other comfort measures and the patient's response.
- Document fluid management, including:
  - intake and output
  - type and size of I.V. catheter
  - location of I.V. line
  - I.V. solution used and flow rate
  - condition of I.V. site.
- Document use of antiembolism stockings, sequential compression device, early ambulation, and prophylactic anticoagulants.
- Include patient education and emotional support given.
- Document drugs given, including:
  - dosage, frequency, and route
  - patient's response.
- If the patient's condition changes, record:
  - name of the doctor notified and time of notification
  - orders received

Memory jogger

When a patient's condition changes, remember **TO DIP** your pen into the chart and document:

Time doctor was notified

Orders received

Doctor's name

Interventions performed

Patient's response to interventions.

– your actions and the patient's response to them.
- Use flow sheets to record:
  – frequent vital signs and assessments
  – intake and output
  – I.V. therapy
  – laboratory values.

12/08/06	1100	Pt. returned from PACU at 1030 S/P laparoscopic laser cholecystectomy. P 88 and regular, BP 112/82, RR 18 deep, regular, tympanic T 98.2° F. Pt. breathing comfortably, breath sounds clear on room air, skin pink and warm, capillary refill less than 3 sec. Sleeping but easily arousable and oriented to time, place, and person. Speech clear and coherent. PERRLA. Normal heart sounds, strong radial and dorsalis pedis pulses bilaterally. Bladder nondistended, no indwelling urinary catheter, doesn't feel urge to void, positive bowel sounds in all 4 quadrants. Abdomen slightly distended, no c/o nausea. Has 4 abdominal puncture wounds covered with 4" X 4" gauze. Dressings without blood or drainage. Pt. c/o of abdominal discomfort rated as 3 on a scale of 0 to 10, w/10 being the worst pain imaginable, refusing analgesics at this time. Pt. placed in semi-Fowler's position, bed in low position, call bell within reach and pt. verbalized understanding of its use. I.V. of 1000 ml $D_5/0.45$ NS infusing at 75 ml/hr in Ⓡ forearm via infusion pump. See flow sheets for documentation of frequent VS, I.V. therapy, and I/O. Explained coughing and deep-breathing exercises to pt. and showed how to splint abdomen with pillow when coughing. Pt. able to give return demo. Told her to call the nurse if she feels she needs pain medication. ———— Gwen Stanz, RN

Preoperative care

- Effective nursing documentation during the preoperative period focuses on the baseline preoperative assessment and patient teaching.
- Documenting these elements encourages accurate communication among caregivers.
- Most facilities use a preoperative checklist to verify that:
  - the required data have been collected and reviewed
  - preoperative teaching has occurred
  - prescribed procedures and safety precautions have been executed
  - site verification has been done.

The write stuff

- Place a check mark in the appropriate column of the preoperative checklist to indicate whether the item has been completed.
- If an item doesn't apply to your patient (such as the use of antiembolism stockings in a patient undergoing a minor surgical procedure), write "N/A."
- When indicated, place your initials in the appropriate column to indicate that an item has been completed.
- Include your full name, credentials, and initials on the form.
- Chart the patient's baseline vital signs on the form.
- Indicate that the procedure site was preoperatively verified according to your facility's standards.
- Before the patient leaves for surgery, check the appropriate boxes to indicate that the patient has been properly and positively identified.
- Document the name of the person you notified of abnormalities that could affect the patient's response to the surgical procedure or deviations from facility standards.

Form fitting

Preoperative checklist

To document preoperative procedures, data collection, and teaching, most facilities use a checklist such as the one below.

Woodview Hospital
Pre-Operative Checklist

Patient name: _Zachary, Timothy_

Medical record number: ___987654___

Instructions: All items checked "No" requires follow up. Follow up is to be documented.
In "Additional Information / Comment" section until resolved.

Pre-Op Checklist	Yes	No	Resolved	Initials
ID Band On	✓			NRC
Allergies Noted / Bracelet	✓			NRC
History & Physical (Present & Reviewed)	✓			NRC
Surgical Informed Consent Signed	✓			NRC
Anesthesia Informed Consent	✓			NRC
Pre-Op Teaching	✓			NRC
Prep. as Ordered	N/A			
NPO After Midnight	✓			NRC
Dentures, Capped Teeth, Cosmetics, Glasses, Contact Lenses, Wig Removed	N/A	✓		
Voided/Catheter Inserted	✓			NRC
Medical Clearance/Physician's Name	✓			NRC
TEDS, as Ordered	N/A			
SCD, as Ordered	N/A			
PCA Teaching, as Ordered	✓			NRC
Type & Cross/Screen Drawn (If Ordered Must Have Blood Informed Consent Signed)	N/A			
**Blood Informed Consent Signed				
*Lab Results on Chart	✓			NRC
*EKG on Chart	✓			NRC
*Chest X-ray on Chart	✓			NRC

*Abnormal Results Results Reported To _H&H Dr. Biletz_

Time & Date _04/28/06   0800_

Reported By _NRC_

Temp. _98.6_ Pulse _84_ Resp. _18_ B/P _132/82_

Valuables

Destination: ☐ To Safe ☐ To Family, Name _____

X _Norma R. Clay, RN_ ___NRC___
Signature of Nurse   Initials

_____

_____

X _____
Signature of Transferring RN   Date   Time

Additional Information /Comments
Pt. has all own teeth

Surgical Patient Identification Form

Nursing Floor RN Patient Identification

☑ Patient I.D. Bracelet Personally Observed
☑ Patient Questioned Verbally Regarding I.D., Procedure & Site
☑ Patient's Chart Reviewed to Verify I.D., Procedure & Site

X _Norma R. Clay, RN_   _04/28/06_   _0800_
R.N.'s Signature   Date   Time

Pre-Op Anesthesia Patient Identification

☐ Patient's I.D. Bracelet Personally Observed
☐ Patient Questioned Verbally Regarding I.D., Procedure & Site
☐ Patient's Chart Reviewed to Verify I.D., Procedure & Site
☐ Surgical Site Marked

X _____
Anesthesiologist/Anesthetist's Signature Date Time

Operating Room and Anesthesia Personnel Patient Identification

Operative Procedure & Site: _____

ANES	CIRC Nurse	
☐	☐	Patient I.D. Bracelet Personally Observed
☐	☐	Patient Questioned Verbally Regarding I.D., Procedure & Site
☐	☐	Patient's Chart Reviewed to Verify I.D., Procedure & Site
☐	☐	Surgical Site Confirmed
☐	☐	**Time-out performed**

X _____
Anesthesiologist/Anesthetist's Signature   Time

X _____
CIRC Nurse's Signature   Time

Surgeon's Patient Identification Statement

☐ Patient I.D. Bracelet Personally Observed
☐ Patient Questioned Verbally Regarding I.D., Procedure & Site
☐ Surgical Site Marked

Pressure ulcer assessment

- Pressure ulcers develop when pressure impairs circulation, depriving tissues of oxygen and life-sustaining nutrients and damaging skin and underlying structures.
- Most pressure ulcers develop over bony prominences, such as the sacrum, coccyx, ischial tuberosities, and greater trochanters, where friction and shearing force combine with pressure to break down skin and underlying tissue.
- In bedridden and immobile patients, pressure ulcers develop over the vertebrae, scapulae, elbows, knees, and heels.
- Untreated pressure ulcers may lead to serious systemic infection.
- Pressure ulcers are staged based on the criteria of the National Pressure Ulcer Advisory Panel and the Agency for Healthcare Research and Quality.
- Determine the patient's risk of developing pressure ulcers using a tool such as the Braden scale, which assesses sensory perception, moisture, activity, mobility, nutrition, and friction and shear.
- Documenting pressure ulcer assessments assists in:
  – identifying at-risk patients
  – reducing the incidence of pressure ulcers
  – monitoring changes in skin condition
  – determining the response to treatment.

The write stuff

- Document the patient's risk factors for pressure ulcer formation, using a tool such as the Braden scale.
- In your note, describe the pressure ulcer, including:
  – its location, size and depth (in centimeters), stage, color, and appearance
  – presence of necrotic or granulation tissue, drainage, and odor

Form fitting

Braden scale: Predicting pressure ulcer risk

The Braden scale, shown below, is the most reliable of several instruments for assessing the older patient's risk of developing pressure ulcers. The lower the score, the greater the risk (15 to 18 = mild risk, 13 or 14 = moderate risk, 10 to 12 = high risk, and ≤ 9 = very high risk).

Patient's name: *Stephin Merritt*   Medical record number: *654321*

Sensory perception Ability to respond meaningfully to pressure-related discomfort	1. Completely limited: Is unresponsive (doesn't moan, flinch, or grasp in response) to painful stimuli because of diminished level of consciousness or sedation OR Has a limited ability to feel pain over most of body surface	2. Very limited: Responds only to painful stimuli; can't communicate discomfort except through moaning or restlessness OR Has a sensory impairment that limits ability to feel pain or discomfort over half of body
Moisture Degree to which skin is exposed to moisture	1. Constantly moist: Skin kept moist almost constantly by perspiration, urine, or other fluids; dampness detected every time patient is moved or turned	2. Very moist: Skin often but not always moist; linen must be changed at least once per shift
Activity Degree of physical activity	1. Bedridden: Confined to bed	2. Chairfast: Ability to walk severely limited or nonexistent; can't bear own weight and must be assisted into chair or wheelchair

Evaluator's name: _James Woodson, RN_

		Date of assessment		
		03/21/06		
3. Slightly limited: Responds to verbal commands but can't always communicate discomfort or need to be turned	4. No impairment: Responds to verbal commands; has no sensory deficit that would limit ability to feel or voice pain or discomfort	3		
3. Occasionally moist: Skin occasionally moist, requiring an extra linen change approximately once per day	4. Rarely moist: Skin usually dry; linen only requires changing at routine intervals	3		
3. Walks occasionally: Walks occasionally during day, but for very short distances, with or without assistance; spends majority of each shift in bed or chair	4. Walks frequently: Walks outside room at least twice per day and inside room at least once every 2 hours during waking hours	2		

(continued)

Braden scale: Predicting pressure ulcer risk *(continued)*

Mobility Ability to change and control body position	1. Completely immobile: Doesn't make even slight changes in body or extremity position without assistance	2. Very limited: Makes occasional slight changes in body or extremity position but is unable to make frequent or significant changes independently
Nutrition Is NPO or maintained on clear liquids or I.V. fluids for more than 5 days	1. Very poor: Never eats a complete meal; rarely eats more than one-third of any food offered; eats two servings or less of protein (meat or dairy products) per day; takes fluids poorly; doesn't take a liquid dietary supplement OR Is NPO or maintained on clear liquids or I.V. fluids for more than 5 days	2. Probably inadequate: Rarely eats a complete meal and generally eats only about half of any food offered; protein intake includes only three servings of meat or dairy products per day; occasionally will take a dietary supplement OR Receives less than optimum amount of liquid diet or tube feeding
Friction and shear Ability to assist with movement or to be moved in a way that prevents skin contact with bedding or other surfaces	1. Problem: Requires moderate to maximum assistance in moving; complete lifting without sliding against sheets is impossible; frequently slides down in bed or chair, requiring frequent repositioning with maximum assistance; spasticity, contractures, or agitation leads to almost constant friction	2. Potential problem: Moves feebly or requires minimum assistance during a move; skin probably slides to some extent against sheets, chair restraints, or other devices; maintains relatively good position in chair or bed most of the time but occasionally slides down

		Date of assessment			
		03/21/06			
3. Slightly limited: Makes frequent though slight changes in body or extremity position independently	4. No limitations: Makes major and frequent changes in body or extremity position without assistance	2			
3. Adequate: Eats more than half of most meals; eats four servings of protein (meat and dairy products) per day; occasionally refuses a meal but will usually take a supplement if offered OR Is on a tube feeding or total parenteral nutrition regimen that probably meets most nutritional needs	4. Excellent: Eats most of every meal and never refuses a meal; usually eats four or more servings of meat and dairy products per day; occasionally eats between meals; doesn't require supplementation	2			
3. No apparent problem: Moves in bed and in chair independently and has sufficient muscle strength to lift up completely during move; maintains good position in bed or chair at all times		2			
	Total	14			

– extent of any undermining
– condition of the surrounding tissue.
- Document the appearance of the pressure ulcer with each dressing change or at least weekly for the patient at home.

01/18/06	1100	Pt. admitted from Green Brier Nursing Home. Pt. has stage 2 pressure ulcer on coccyx, approx. 2 cm X 1 cm X 0.5 cm. No drainage noted. Base has deep pink granulation tissue. Skin surrounding ulcer pink, intact, well-defined edges. Ulcer covered with transparent dressing. Braden score 14 (see Braden Pressure Ulcer Risk Assessment Scale). —————————— James Woodson, RN

Pressure ulcer care

- Pressure ulcer treatment involves:
  - relieving pressure
  - restoring circulation
  - promoting healing
  - managing related disorders.
- The effectiveness and duration of treatment depend on the pressure ulcer's characteristics.
- Prevention is the key to avoiding extensive therapy and includes ensuring adequate nourishment and mobility to relieve pressure and promote circulation.
- When a pressure ulcer develops despite preventive efforts, treatment includes:
  - frequent repositioning to shorten pressure duration
  - use of special equipment to reduce pressure intensity.
- Other therapeutic measures include risk-factor reduction and the use of topical treatments, wound cleansing, debridement, and dressings to support moist wound healing.
- When caring for a wound, always follow the standard precautions guidelines of the Centers for Disease Control and Prevention.

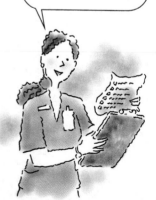

Preventing pressure ulcers is a primary goal, so be sure to chart preventive measures used.

The write stuff

- Record the date and time of dressing changes and treatments.
- Note the specific treatment and the patient's response.
- Detail preventive strategies performed.

- Document the pressure ulcer's:
  - location and size (length, width, and depth in centimeters)
  - color and appearance of the wound bed
  - amount, color, odor, and consistency of drainage
  - condition of surrounding skin.
- Reassess ulcers with each dressing change and at least weekly.
- Note changes in:
  - condition or size of the pressure ulcer
  - skin temperature.
- Document:
  - name of the practitioner notified of ulcer changes
  - time of notification
  - orders received.
- Record the patient's temperature on the graphic sheet to allow easy assessment of temperature patterns.
- Chart patient education, such as:
  - your explanation of treatments
  - the need for turning and positioning every 2 hours
  - proper nutrition.
- Update the care plan as required.

04/20/06	1230	Pt. has stage 2 pressure ulcer on Ⓛ heel.
		Approx. 2 cm X 5 cm X 1 cm. Base of ulcer has
		necrotic tissue, no drainage. Skin around ulcer
		intact. P 82, BP 134/78, RR 18, oral T 98.6° F.
		Wet-to-dry dressing removed and ulcer
		irrigated with NSS. Gauze moistened with NSS,
		placed in wound bed, and covered with dry
		sterile 4" X 4" gauze. Pt. turned and
		repositioned. Heels elevated off bed with
		pillow placed lengthwise under legs. Dietitian
		in to see pt. High-protein, high-calorie shakes
		being encouraged with each meal. Explained
		importance of proper nutrition for wound
		healing. ——————— Harriet Newman, RN

Pulmonary edema

- Pulmonary edema is a diffuse extravascular accumulation of fluid in the tissues and airspaces of the lungs due to increased pressure in the pulmonary capillaries.
- It can be a chronic condition, or it can develop quickly and rapidly become life-threatening. If your patient shows signs of pulmonary edema, notify the practitioner immediately.
- Administer oxygen by nasal cannula or facemask for hypoxemia. Also position the patient to facilitate breathing, such as high Fowler's position.
- If respiratory distress develops, prepare for intubation and mechanical ventilation.
- Administer drugs as ordered, such as diuretics, nitrates, morphine, inotropics, vasodilators, and angiotensin-converting enzyme inhibitors.
- Anticipate assisting with the insertion of hemodynamic monitoring lines.
- Reassure the patient and family, and explain procedures.

The write stuff

- Record the date and time of your entry.
- Document your assessment findings of pulmonary edema, such as dyspnea or tachypnea; pink, frothy sputum; and adventitious or diminished breath sounds.
- Note:
  - name of the practitioner notified and time of notification
  - orders received (such as oxygen and drug administration and chest X-ray).
- Record your interventions, such as:
  - positioning the patient in high Fowler's position, with legs dangling
  - inserting I.V. lines
  - administering oxygen and drugs
  - assisting with hemodynamic monitoring line insertion
  - suctioning.

- Chart the patient's responses to interventions.
- Use flow sheets to record:
  - frequent vital signs and assessments
  - hemodynamic measurements
  - intake and output
  - I.V. therapy
  - laboratory test and arterial blood gas values.
- Include patient teaching and emotional care given.

09/17/06	0300	Pt. discovered lying flat in bed at 0230 trying to sit up and stating, "I can't breathe." Pt. coughing and bringing up small amount of pink, frothy sputum. Skin pale, lips cyanotic, sluggish capillary refill, +1 ankle edema bilaterally. Lungs with crackles halfway up bilaterally, S_3 heard on auscultation of heart. P 120 and irregular, BP 140/90, RR 30 and shallow, tympanic T 98.8° F. Pt. restless, alert, and oriented to time, place, and person. Dr. Clooney notified of assessment findings at 0235 and came to see pt. at 0245. Pt. placed in sitting position with legs dangling. O_2 via NC at 2 L/min changed to nonrebreather mask at 12 L/min. Explained to pt. that mask would give her more O_2 and help her breathing. O_2 sat. by pulse oximetry 81%. Stat portable CXR done. 12-lead ECG shows sinus tachycardia with occasional PVCs. CBC and electrolytes drawn and sent to lab stat. Morphine, furosemide, and digoxin I.V. ordered and given through intermittent infusion device in ® forearm. See MAR. Indwelling urinary catheter inserted to straight drainage, drained 100 ml on insertion. Pt. encouraged to cough and deep-breathe. Explained all procedures and drugs to pt. Reassured pt. that she's being closely monitored. See flow sheets for documentation of frequent VS, I/O, and lab values. — Rachel Moreau, R.N

Pulse oximetry

- Pulse oximetry is a noninvasive procedure used to monitor a patient's arterial blood oxygen saturation (SpO_2) to detect hypoxemia.
- Lack of adequate oxygenation can cause permanent cellular damage and death.
- A sensor containing two light-emitting diodes (LEDs)—one red and one infrared—and a photodetector placed opposite these LEDs across a vascular bed are attached to the skin with adhesive or clips.
- The sensor is placed across a pulsating arteriolar bed, such as a finger, toe, nose, or earlobe.
- Selected wavelengths of light are absorbed by hemoglobin and transmitted through tissue to the photodetector.
- The pulse oximeter computes SpO_2 based on the relative amounts of light that reach the photodetector with the normal value being between 95% and 100%.
- Pulse oximetry may be performed intermittently or continuously.

The write stuff

- Record the date and time of each pulse oximetry reading.
- Frequent SpO_2 readings may be documented on a flow sheet.
- Document the reason for use of pulse oximetry and whether readings are continuous or intermittent.
- If SpO_2 readings are continuous, record the alarm settings.
- Document whether the reading is obtained while the patient is breathing room air or receiving supplemental oxygen.
- If the patient is receiving oxygen, record the concentration and mode of delivery.
- Describe events precipitating acute oxygen desaturation, your actions, and the patient's response.
- Record activities or interventions affecting SpO_2 values.
- Document patient teaching related to pulse oximetry.

03/13/06	1100	At 1040 pt. dyspneic with c/o SOB. P 128, BP 140/96, RR 34, tympanic T 97.3° F. Lips and nail beds cyanotic. Lungs clear. Able to speak only 2 or 3 words between breaths due to dyspnea. O_2 NC resting on bedside table. Pt.'s wife Sue states, "He took it off because it hurts his ears." Pulse oximetry 86%. NC reapplied at 6 L/min. Pt. less dyspneic, able to speak in sentences. P 100, BP 136/90, RR 26. Pt. monitored on continuous pulse oximetry. O_2 sat 93% at 1045. Pt. and wife instructed to leave NC in place in nostrils. Tubing padded around earpieces for comfort. Pt. instructed to call the nurse if tubing becomes uncomfortable rather than removing it. Pt. and wife verbalized understanding of the need for the oximetry monitoring. ———————— *Lesley Alexander, RN*

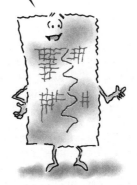

Frequent SpO_2 readings may be documented on a flow sheet.

R-Z

Regulatory agencies and patient safety goals provide standards for charting and keep you and your patient in the safe zone.

D-H

O-Q

R-Z

Misc.

R

Rape trauma

- The term *rape* refers to nonconsensual sexual intercourse.
- Rape-trauma syndrome occurs following the rape or attempted rape and refers to the:
  - victim's short- and long-term reactions
  - methods the victim uses to cope with the trauma.
- Be objective when documenting care for a rape victim; your notes may be used as evidence if the rapist is tried.

The write stuff

- Record the date and time of each entry.
- Chart the patient's statements, using her own words, in quotes.
- Include:
  - time the patient arrived at the facility
  - date and time of the alleged rape
  - time that the patient was examined.
- Document that the patient gave consent for treatment.
- Document:
  - allergies to penicillin and other drugs
  - recent illnesses (especially venereal disease)
  - possibility of pregnancy before the attack
  - date of her last menses
  - details of her obstetric and gynecologic history.
- Describe the patient's emotional state and behaviors.
- Note whether the patient douched or washed since the rape.
- Label all specimens with:
  - patient's name
  - practitioner's name
  - location from which the specimen was obtained.
- List all specimens in your notes; include the name of the person to whom they were given.

- Document whether photographs were taken.
- Note the name of any counselor present.
- Chart all medications given, such as antibiotics and birth control prophylaxis, on the medication administration record.
- Record care given to any injuries.
- Document testing, such as for human immunodeficiency virus or hepatitis B and C, and whether prophylaxis for hepatitis was given.
- Chart that you told the patient the importance of follow-up testing in 5 to 6 days for gonorrhea and syphilis.
- Record that contact information for such services as rape crisis centers, victims' rights advocates, and local law enforcement was given to the patient.
- Chart education and support given to the patient.

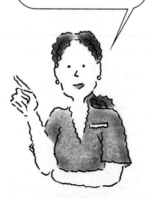

Specimens obtained from a rape victim need to be labeled with the patient's name, practitioner's name, and location from which they were obtained.

08/10/06	2250	Pt. brought to ED by police officers Dale Cooper (badge #1234) and Tom Collins (badge #5678). Pt. states, "I was raped in the supermarket parking lot." Pt. crying but able to walk into ED on her own. Placed in private room. Pt. denies pregnancy, allergies, and recent illnesses. LMP 7/28/06. States she didn't wash or douche since attack. After explaining procedure, Dr. Hayward examined pt. Pt. has reddened areas on anterior neck. Bruising noted on inner aspects of both thighs; some vaginal bleeding. See dr.'s note for details of pelvic exam. Specimens for VD, blood, and vaginal smears collected and labeled. Evidence from fingernail scraping and pubic hair combing collected and labeled. Chain of evidence maintained. Photographs taken of injuries. Ceftriaxone 250 mg I.M. given in ① dorsogluteal muscle. Pt. declined morning-after pill. Pt. consented to screening for HIV and hepatitis. Blood samples drawn, labeled, and sent to lab. Pt. understands need for f/u tests for HIV, hepatitis, and VD ——— ————————————— Laura Palmer, RN
08/10/06	2330	Madeleine Ferguson, MSW, spoke with pt. at length. Gave pt. information on rape crisis center and victims' rights advocate. Pt. states, "I'll call them. Ms. Ferguson told me they can help me deal with this." Pt. phoned brother, who will come to hospital and take pt. to his home for the night. Police officers interviewed pt. with her permission regarding the details of the event. At pt.'s request, Ms. Ferguson and myself remained with her. Laura Palmer, RN
08/10/06	2350	Pt.'s brother, Pete Martell, and his wife, Catherine Martell, arrived to take pt. to their house. Pt. will make appt. tomorrow to f/u with own dr. next week or sooner, if needed. Pt. has names and phone numbers for rape crisis counselor, victims' rights advocate, Ms. Ferguson, ED, and police dept. ——— Laura Palmer, RN

Refusal of treatment

- Any mentally competent adult can refuse treatment.
- In most cases, health care personnel can remain free from legal jeopardy as long as they fully inform the patient about his medical condition and the likely consequences of refusing treatment and follow through with any medical and laboratory tests that have been initiated.
- The courts recognize a competent adult's right to refuse medical treatment, even when that refusal will clearly lead to his death.
- When your patient refuses treatment, inform him of the risks involved in making such a decision.
- If possible, inform the patient in writing.
- If he continues to refuse treatment, notify the practitioner, who will choose the most appropriate plan of action, and the nursing supervisor.
- The courts recognize several situations that justify overruling a patient's refusal of treatment, such as when:
  – refusing treatment endangers the life of another

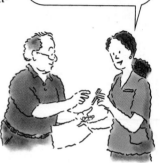

Refusing treatment at this time? Fine. Just sign on the dotted line.

Making a case

Respecting a patient's right to refuse care

Never ignore a patient's request to refuse treatment. A patient can sue you for battery—intentionally touching another person without authorization—for simply following a practitioner's orders.

To overrule the patient's decision, the practitioner or your facility must obtain a court order. Only then are you legally authorized to administer the treatment.

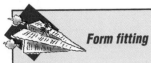

Form fitting

Refusal of treatment form

REFUSAL OF TREATMENT RELEASE FORM

I, _____Keith Nelson_____ , refuse to allow anyone to
 [patient's name]

perform tests to diagnose heart attack & treat for heart attack .
 [insert treatment]

The risks attendant to my refusal have been fully explained to me, and I fully understand the results for this treatment and that if the same isn't done, my chances for regaining my normal health are seriously reduced and that, in all probability, my refusal for such treatment or procedure will seriously affect my health or recovery.

I hereby release _____Memorial Hospital_____ ,
 [name of hospital]

its nurses and employees, together with all doctors in any way connected with me as a patient, from liability for respecting and following my expressed wishes and direction.

Amanda Jones, RN	_Keith Nelson_
Witness	Patient or Legal Guardian
_01/23/06_	_03/05/58_
Date	Patient's date of birth

- a parent's decision threatens a child's life
- despite refusing treatment, the patient makes statements indicating he wants to live.
• Have the patient sign a refusal of treatment form indicating appropriate treatment would have been given had the patient consented.

The write stuff
• Record the date and time of your entry.

- Document that you explained the care and the risks involved in not receiving it.
- Document your patient's understanding of the risks, using his own words.
- Record the names of the nursing supervisor and practitioner you notified and the time of notification.
- Document that the practitioner saw the patient and explained the risks of refusing treatment.
- Chart whether the patient signed a refusal of treatment form.
- If the patient refuses to sign the refusal form:
  - write "refused to sign" in the space for the patient's signature
  - place your initials and date beside it
  - document his refusal to sign in your nurse's note.
- Document that you didn't provide the prescribed treatment because the patient refused it.
- If your facility's policy requires you to ask the patient's spouse or closest relative to sign another refusal of treatment release form, document which relative signs the form.

09/08/06	2000	Pt. refusing to have I.V. line inserted, stating that he's "sick and tired of being stuck." Explained to pt. the need for I.V. fluids and antibiotics and the likely result of refusing treatment. Dr. Fitzgerald notified at 1930 and came to see pt. Dr. Fitzgerald spent 20 minutes with pt. explaining rationales for therapies and potential risks of refusing therapy. Pt. still refusing I.V. line. Pt. has agreed to drink at least 4 oz of fluid every hour and take oral antibiotics. Pt. verbalized understanding that oral antibiotics aren't as effective in treating his condition. Orders written for 4 oz of fluids P.O. qlhr; amoxicillin 250 mg P.O. q8hr. Repeat electrolytes in a.m. ———————————— William Bard, RN

Reports to practitioner

- Reports you need to communicate to the practitioner within a reasonable time frame are included in *Patient Safety Goals* and include:
  - changes in the patient's condition
  - abnormal laboratory and other critical test results
  - patient concerns.
- Proper and timely reporting and documentation of reports to the practitioner are essential.
  - You may be noncompliant meeting standards when reporting and documentation aren't timely.
  - If a patient's care comes into question, the practitioner could claim that he wasn't notified.
  - Writing "Notified practitioner of lab results" is too vague.
  - In the event of a malpractice suit, it allows the plaintiff's lawyer (and the practitioner) to imply that you didn't communicate reports to the practitioner or there was a delay in reporting.

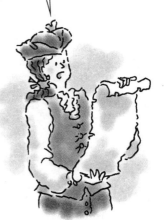

Whether it's by phone, fax, or town cryer, document what means you used to communicate a report to the practitioner.

The write stuff

- Record the date and time you notified the practitioner and the practitioner's name.
- Chart the means you used to communicate and what you reported. A critical result must not be faxed.

- If you left a message for the practitioner or gave a result to someone else, such as a receptionist, record that person's name as well. Critical results must be verbally given to a responsible caregiver.
- Record the practitioner's response and any orders received.
- If no orders are received, document that as well.

09/13/06	2215	Called Dr. Spencer at 2200 to report increased serous drainage from pt.'s ⓛ chest tube. Dr. Spencer's order was to observe the drainage for 1 more hr and then call him back. ——————————————————— Shelly Johnson, RN

Respiratory arrest

- Respiratory arrest is defined as loss of consciousness due to the absence of respirations sufficient to provide adequate oxygenation.
- If a patient is found unresponsive without adequate respirations, rapid intervention is critical because brain death may occur within minutes after respirations cease.
  - Immediately call for help and send a coworker to call the code team and the practitioner.
  - Open the airway and assess the patient's breathing.
  - If absent, begin rescue breathing (using a pocket face-mask) and cardiopulmonary resuscitation (CPR), according to the American Heart Association guidelines.
  - Continue until respirations return spontaneously and are sufficient for adequate oxygenation or ventilatory support via endotracheal (ET) intubation and mechanical ventilation can be instituted.
- Most facilities use a code sheet to facilitate documentation of respiratory arrest.

The write stuff

- Use your facility's code sheet to record:
  - date and time that the patient was found unresponsive and without respirations
  - name of the person who found the patient
  - whether the event was witnessed
  - name of the person who initiated CPR and the time CPR was initiated
  - names of the other members of the code team
  - signatures of all members of the code team
  - interventions performed (such as drugs administered, cardiac monitoring, ET intubation, and arterial blood gas analysis), the time they occurred, and the patient's response

- outcome of the code (for example, whether the patient resumed spontaneous respirations, received mechanical ventilation, or expired)
- whether the family was present or the time the family was notified of the event.
- In your narrative note, include:
  - events leading to the respiratory arrest
  - assessment findings prompting you to call a code
  - other interventions performed before the code team arrived (such as the time that CPR was initiated and who initiated it)
  - patient's response to the interventions
  - that a code sheet was used to document the events of the code.

| 10/03/06 | 1440 | Found pt. unresponsive on floor next to his bed at 1428. Airway opened using head-tilt, chin-lift maneuver; no respirations noted. Called for help. Lucy Moran, RN, arrived and was sent to call code team at 1431. Ventilation attempt via pocket facemask unsuccessful. Head repositioned but still unable to deliver breath. No foreign bodies noted in mouth. After delivery of 3rd abdominal thrust, piece of meat was expelled. Pt. still without respirations; carotid pulse palpable. Rescue breathing initiated via facemask. Code team arrived at 1433 and continued resuscitative efforts. See code record. _Josie Packard, R.N_ |
| 10/03/06 | 1450 | Pt. resumed respirations and opened eyes. P 68, BP 102/52, RR 32 unlabored and deep. Placed on O_2 2 L/min via NC. Pt. being transferred to ICU for observation. Report called to Shelly Johnson, RN, at 1445. Family notified of pt.'s condition and transfer to ICU. Family will call ICU in 1 hour to check on pt.'s condition. ——— _Josie Packard, R.N_ |

Respiratory distress

- Respiratory distress occurs when abnormalities of oxygenation or carbon dioxide are severe enough to endanger the function of vital organs.
- Causes of respiratory distress may be pulmonary or nonpulmonary in origin and may include a failure of oxygenation, ventilation, or both.
- Common causes of respiratory distress include pulmonary edema, pulmonary embolism, asthma, chronic obstructive pulmonary disease, and sedative and opioid overmedication.
- Respiratory distress can develop gradually or suddenly and can quickly become a life-threatening emergency.
- If your patient develops respiratory distress, initiate oxygen administration and notify the practitioner immediately.
- Anticipate interventions, such as:
  - chest X-ray
  - mobilizing secretions
  - initiating endotracheal (ET) intubation and mechanical ventilation
  - administering drug therapy to relieve bronchospasm, reduce airway inflammation, and alleviate severe anxiety and restlessness.

The write stuff

- Record the date and time of your entry.
- Record your assessment findings of respiratory distress, such as dyspnea, abnormal breath sounds, restlessness, and confusion.

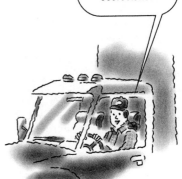

- Note:
  - name of the practitioner notified
  - time of notification
  - orders received, such as oxygen and drug administration.
- Record your interventions, such as:
  - obtaining a chest X-ray
  - inserting I.V. lines
  - administering oxygen and drugs
  - monitoring pulse oximetry and arterial blood gas (ABG) studies
  - assisting with the insertion of hemodynamic monitoring lines
  - assisting with ET intubation
  - maintaining mechanical ventilation
  - suctioning.
- Document the patient's responses to interventions.
- Use flow sheets to record:
  - frequent assessments
  - vital signs
  - hemodynamic measurements
  - intake and output
  - I.V. therapy
  - laboratory and ABG values.
- Document education and emotional support given to the patient and his family.

06/05/06	1500	At 1430 while receiving mechlorethamine via
		implanted port, pt. c/o chills and reported, "I
		have tightness in my chest. It feels like my
		throat is closing up." Drug infusion stopped
		and NSS infusing at 20 ml/hr. Pt. dyspneic,
		diaphoretic, and restless. P 122 and regular,
		BP 169/90, RR 34. O₂ sat. by pulse oximetry
		88%. Expiratory wheezes noted bilaterally on
		posterior and anterior chest auscultation.
		Accessory muscle use observed. Dr. Hurley stat
		paged at 1437 and told of assessment
		findings. orders received. Nonrebreather mask
		applied at 12 L/minute. Pt. placed in tripod
		position to facilitate breathing. Stat ABGs
		drawn by Dr. Hurley. I.V. methylprednisolone
		given. See MAR. At 1450 P 104, BP 140/84, RR
		30. Pulse oximetry 95%. Pt. states her
		breathing is easier, no further chills. Breath
		sounds clear, no longer using accessory
		muscles. See flow sheets for documentation of
		frequent VS, I/O, and lab values. Reassured
		pt. that she will be closely monitored. ————
		————————————— Angela Badalamenti, RN

Restraint use

- Restraints are defined as any method of physically restricting a person's freedom of movement, physical activity, or normal access to his body.
- According to the standards issued by the Joint Commission on Accreditation of Healthcare Organizations (JCAHO) regarding the use of restraints on the medical-surgical unit, restraint use is to be limited to emergencies in which the patient is at risk for harming himself or others.
- JCAHO standards also emphasize staff education; know and follow your facility's policy on the use of restraints.
- Within 12 hours of placing a patient in restraints, a practitioner must give an order for restraints; however, if the need for restraints is due to a significant change in the patient's condition, the nurse must notify the practitioner immediately.
- JCAHO standards require monitoring to ensure patient safety, including monitoring the patient's vital signs, and meeting nutrition, hydration, circulation, and hygiene and toileting needs according to facility policy.
- The patient's family must be notified of the use of restraints if the patient consented to have them informed of his care.
- The patient must be informed of the conditions necessary for his release from restraints.

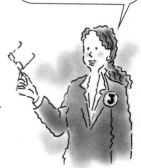

Proper documentation of restraint use provides evidence of your compliance with JCAHO standards.

Form fitting

Restraint and safety device flow sheet

RESTRAINT AND SAFETY DEVICE FLOW SHEET

Patient name: *Jack Mickelson*
Medical record #: *13/3/3*

1. Physician ordering:
   Dr. Curley
   Date: *09/02/06* Time: *1400*
2. Type of restraint: *® & ® soft wrist restraints*
3. Behavior requiring restraint: _____
   Patient extremely confused, pulled out I.V.

Legend

Time	0000	0200	0400	0600	0800	1000
Skin/ Circulation						
Range of motion						
Position						
Fluid/ Nourishment/ Toilet offered						
Vital signs						
Readiness for restraint removal						
Safety checks						

4. Interventions attempted:

Diversion with TV

Education

Covering I.V. site with Ace

wrap

5. Restraint use explanation given to:
   ☐ Patient
   ☐ Family
   ☐ Guardian

6. Document assessment/activity every 2 hours. Circle and describe variations in narrative notes:

1200	1400	1600	1800	2000	2200
	ℝ & 𝕃 radial pulse strong, cap refill < 3 sec., skin intact, hands warm, pink				
	AROM to ℝ & 𝕃 arms				
	Turned from ℝ to 𝕃 side				
	Drank 240 ml juice, declined snack, voided				
	P 88, RR 18, BP 122/64, T 97.2 axillary				
	Continues pulling at I.V. tubing				
	TJ TJ				

Initials   Signature

_T.J_   _Tom Jones, RN_

The write stuff

- Document each episode of the use of restraints, including the date and time they were initiated.
- Use a special form, if required by your facility.
- Record:
  - circumstances leading to the use of restraints
  - nonphysical interventions considered or used first.
- Describe the rationale for the specific type of restraints used.
- Document the name of the practitioner who ordered the restraints.
- Include the conditions or behaviors necessary for discontinuing the restraints and that these conditions were communicated to the patient.
- Document each in-person evaluation by the practitioner.
- Record that you checked on the patient on initiation of restraint use and every 2 hours thereafter.
- Record 2-hour assessments of the patient, including:
  - signs of injury
  - nutrition, hydration, circulation, range of motion, elimination, comfort, hygiene, physical, and psychological status
  - vital signs
  - readiness for removing the restraints.
- Record your interventions to help the patient meet the conditions for removing the restraints.
- Note that the patient was monitored as needed and according to facility policy.

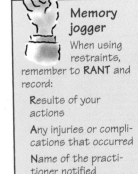

Memory jogger

When using restraints, remember to **RANT** and record:

Results of your actions

Any injuries or complications that occurred

Name of the practitioner notified

Time of occurrence.

- Document any injuries or complications that occurred, the time they occurred, the name of the practitioner notified, and the results of your interventions or actions.

08/28/06	1400	Pt. extremely confused and pulled I.V. out at
		1345. Attempted to calm patient through
		nonthreatening verbal communication. No I.V.
		access available. Dr. Lynch notified at 1350 and
		came to see pt. at 1353. Ativan 2 mg I.M.
		given per Dr. Lynch's order. After evaluation,
		Dr. Lynch ordered 2-point restraints applied
		to prevent harm to patient. Pt. informed that
		restraints would be removed when he could
		remain calm and refrain from trying to
		remove I.V. Pt. doesn't want his family to be
		notified of restraint application. See restraint
		monitoring sheet for frequent assessments
		and intervention notations. ——— Jack Nance, RN

S

Search of patient or belongings

- The fourth amendment to the Constitution protects individuals from unreasonable searches of their person, house, office, or vehicle.
- A search is justified when there are reasonable grounds to believe that the search will produce evidence of a violation of the law or rules of the institution.
- It's generally accepted that the police may not enter a person's home without a search warrant; typically, this guideline also applies to the patient's hospital room.
- If a patient's belongings are to be searched by law enforcement authorities, immediately notify the:
  - nursing supervisor
  - facility administrator
  - legal affairs department.
- Don't allow search or seizure until you've ensured that the patient's legal rights are protected and the law enforcement agency that would like to perform the search has presented a search warrant.
- The facility is required to cooperate with law enforcement agencies in the collection and preservation of evidence involving patients, in accordance with appropriate medical ethics and legal statutes.

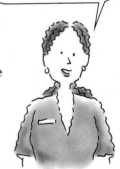

Protect your patient's rights during a search. Make sure a warrant is presented and document that it was done.

The write stuff

- Record the date and time of your entry.
- Document that a search warrant was presented by law enforcement agents, including:
  - time of the presentation of the search warrant
  - names of the nursing supervisor, hospital administrator, and practitioner who witnessed the presentation.
- Record the rationale for searching the patient's belongings.
- Document compliance with your facility's and local law enforcement's policies and procedures before instituting the search.
- Record:
  - time that the search occurred
  - name of the person conducting the search
  - names of others present.

06/22/06	1700	Presented with search warrant by police officers
		J. Friday (badge #1234) and P. Streebeck
		(badge #5678) at 1630 to search patient's
		belongings for crime evidence. Notified Connie
		Swail, RN, nursing supervisor; Alan White,
		hospital administrator; and Dr. Chaddha of
		search warrant at 1635. Ms. Swail and Mr.
		White arrived on unit at 1640 to review
		search warrant. Search took place at 1645 by
		officers Friday and Streebeck, with Ms. Swail,
		Mr. White, and I in attendance. Yellow watch,
		brown wallet, and yellow necklace with clear
		stone removed from pt.'s jacket. ————
		—————————— Tammy Hanks, RN

Shock

- Shock is characterized by diffuse cellular ischemia that leads to cell, tissue, and organ death if not promptly treated.
- Shock is classified as:
  - hypovolemic
  - cardiogenic
  - distributive.
- Distributive shock is further divided into:
  - septic
  - neurogenic
  - anaphylactic.
- Shock is typically treated in an intensive care unit.
- Nursing responsibilities center on prevention, early detection, emergency treatment, and support during recovery and rehabilitation.

The write stuff

- Record the date and time of your entry.
- Document assessment findings, such as declining level of consciousness, hypotension, tachycardia, declining arterial oxygen saturation, and oliguria.
- Note:
  - name of the practitioner notified
  - time of notification
  - orders received.
- Record your interventions, such as:
  - assisting with the insertion of hemodynamic monitoring lines
  - infusing I.V. fluids
  - administering drugs
  - continuous electrocardiogram monitoring
  - providing supplemental oxygen
  - inserting an indwelling urinary catheter
  - airway management
  - pulse oximetry monitoring.

Types of shock

Type	Description
Hypovolemic	• Shock results from a decrease in central vascular volume. • Total body fluids may or may not be decreased. • Causes include hemorrhage, dehydration, and fluid shifts (trauma, burns, anaphylaxis).
Cardiogenic	• Shock results from a direct or indirect pump failure with decreasing cardiac output. • Total body fluid isn't decreased. • Causes include valvular stenosis or insufficiency, myocardial infarction, cardiomyopathy, arrhythmias, cardiac arrest, cardiac tamponade, pericarditis, pulmonary hypertension, and pulmonary emboli.
Distributive	• Shock results from inadequate vascular tone that leads to massive vasodilation. • Vascular volume remains normal and heart pumps adequately, but size of vascular space increases, causing maldistribution of blood within the circulatory system.
Septic	• This subtype is a form of severe sepsis characterized by hypotension and altered tissue perfusion. • Vascular tone is lost and cardiac output may be decreased.
Neurogenic	• This subtype type is characterized by massive vasodilation from loss or suppression of sympathetic tone. • Causes include head trauma, spinal cord injuries, anesthesia, and stress.
Anaphylactic	• This subtype is characterized by massive vasodilation and increased capillary permeability secondary to a hypersensitivity reaction to an antigen.

- Document the patient's responses to interventions.
- Use flow sheets to record:
  - frequent assessments
  - vital signs
  - hemodynamic measurements
  - intake and output
  - I.V. therapy
  - laboratory test and arterial blood gas values.
- Record teaching and emotional care given.

| 07/17/06 | 1930 | At 1905, noted bloody abdominal dressing and abdominal distention. No bowel sounds auscultated. Pt. slow to respond to verbal stimulation, not oriented to time and place, and not readily following commands. Pupil response sluggish. Cardiac monitor reveals HR of 128, no arrhythmias noted. Peripheral pulses weak. Skin pale and cool; capillary refill 4-5 sec, BP 88/52. Breath sounds clear. Normal heart sounds. Breathing regular and deep, RR 24. O₂ sat. 88% on room air. Dr. Garcia notified of changes at 1910 and orders received. 100% nonrebreather mask applied, O₂ sat. increased to 92%. Foley catheter placed with initial 70 ml urine output. Stat ABG, hemoglobin, hematocrit, serum electrolytes and renal panel ordered. I.V. inserted in ℝ antecubital space with 18G catheter on first attempt. 1000 ml I.V. dextrose 5% in 0.45% NSS infusing at 100 ml/hr. Explained all procedures and drugs to pt. and wife. Wife verbalized understanding and fears. Reassured wife that pt. is being closely monitored. See flow sheets for documentation of frequent VS, I/O, I.V. fluids, neuro. checks, and lab values. ———————— Brian Wilson, RN |

Skin care

- In addition to helping shape a patient's self-image, skin has several physiologic functions.
    - It protects internal body structures from the environment and potential pathogens.
    - It regulates body temperature and homeostasis.
    - It serves as an organ of sensation and excretion.
- Meticulous skin care is essential to overall health.

The write stuff

- Record the date and time of your entry.
- Chart the condition of your patient's skin, noting changes in color, temperature, texture, tone, turgor, thickness, moisture, and integrity.
- Describe your interventions related to skin care, such as turning and repositioning the patient every 2 hours, wound care, and monitoring risk of pressure ulcers.
- Record the patient's response to your nursing interventions.
- Document:
    - name of the practitioner notified of any skin changes
    - time of notification
    - orders received
    - actions taken
    - patient's response.
- Include patient teaching provided, such as:
    - proper hygiene
    - importance of turning and repositioning every 2 hours.

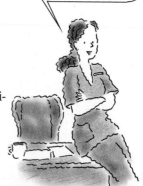

Meticulous skin care is an important part of overall health. Be sure to document it!

12/22/06	1000	During a.m. care, noted pt.'s skin to be dry and flaking, especially the hands, feet, and lower legs. Pt. states skin feels itchy in these areas. Skin rough, intact, warm to touch. Skin tents when pinched. After bath, blotted skin dry and applied emollient. Explained the importance of drinking more fluids and using emollients. Encouraged pt. not to scratch skin and to report intense itching to nurse. Care plan amended to include use of superfatted soap with baths and application of emollients t.i.d. Dr. Baxter notified at 0945 and order received for Benadryl 0.25 mg P.O. q6hr prn for intense itching. Pt. states, "The itching is not bad now that the cream was applied." ———————————— Gil Shepherd, RN

Stat drug administration order

- A drug that's ordered stat is to be administered to the patient immediately for an urgent medical problem.
- This single-dose medication should be documented in the medication administration record (MAR) and in the progress notes.

The write stuff

- Record the date and time of your entry.
- Document:
  - name of the practitioner who gave the order
  - why the order was given
  - patient's response to the drug.
- In the MAR, write:
  - drug's name
  - dosage
  - route
  - time given.

02/03/07	0900	Pt. SOB, with crackles auscultated bilaterally in the bases and O_2 sat. decreased to 89% on room air. P 104, BP 92/60, RR 32 and labored. Lasix 40 mg P.O. given per Dr. Weston's order.
		———————————— Hope Steadman, RN
02/03/07	1000	Pt. responded with urine output of 1500 ml, decreased SOB, and O_2 sat. increased to 97% on room air. P 98, BP 94/60, and RR 28. ———
		———————————— Hope Steadman, RN

Status asthmaticus

- An acute, life-threatening obstructive lung disorder, status asthmaticus doesn't respond to conventional asthma therapy and requires more aggressive treatment.
- Uncontrolled, status asthmaticus can lead to respiratory arrest or heart failure.
- Status asthmaticus may be triggered by allergens, occupational and environmental irritants, infections such as pneumonia, cold weather, and exercise.
- If your patient's asthma continues to worsen despite medical treatment, suspect status asthmaticus and call the practitioner immediately.
- Anticipate:
  - administration of inhaled beta$_2$-adrenergic or anticholinergic drugs, subcutaneous (subQ) epinephrine, I.V. aminophylline, corticosteroids, and fluids
  - oxygen administration
  - endotracheal (ET) intubation and mechanical ventilation.

The write stuff

- Record the date and time of your entry.
- Document your assessment findings, such as severe dyspnea, tachycardia, restlessness, wheezes, low arterial oxygen saturation, stridor, or cyanosis.
- Document:
  - name of practitioner notified
  - time of notification
  - orders received, such as drug and fluid administration or oxygen therapy.

- As needed, include:
  - name of the respiratory therapist notified
  - time of notification
  - actions performed
  - patient's response.
- Record your interventions, such as:
  - administering inhaled, I.V., and subQ drugs
  - administering oxygen
  - providing I.V. fluids
  - placing the patient in an upright position
  - calming the patient
  - assisting with ET intubation and mechanical ventilation.
- Chart the patient's response to interventions.
- Use flow sheets to record:
  - frequent assessments
  - frequent vital signs
  - intake and output
  - I.V. therapy
  - laboratory test and arterial blood gas values.
- Include patient teaching and emotional support given.

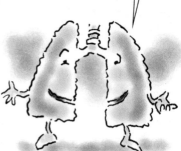

Documenting status asthmaticus is as easy as ABG!

12/13/06	0955	Called to room at 0930 and found pt. severely
		dyspneic stating, "I'm . . . suffocating . . ." Unable
		to speak more than one word at a time.
		Anxious facial expression, using nasal flaring
		and accessory muscles to breathe, restless
		and moving around in bed, skin pale. P 112 and
		regular, BP 142/88, RR 32 and labored.
		Wheezes audible without stethoscope, heard in
		all lung fields on auscultation. O_2 sat. 87%.
		Pt. placed in high Fowler's position and 35%
		oxygen by facemask applied. Called Dr. Murdock
		at 0937 and reported assessment findings.
		Orders received by Dr. Murdock. Stat ABG
		drawn at 0945 by Ted Striker, RRT. I.V. line
		started on first attempt with #22G angiocath
		in ® hand. 1000 ml NSS infusing at 100
		ml/hr. Methylprednisolone 150 mg given I.V.P.
		Nebulized albuterol administered by Mr. Striker.
		Stayed with pt. throughout event, explaining all
		procedures and offering reassurances. See
		flow sheets for documentation of frequent VS,
		I/O, I.V., and ABG values. ————————
		———————————— Lesley Neilsen, RN
12/13/06	1010	ABG results: pH 7.33, PaO_2 75 mm Hg, $PaCO_2$
		50 mm Hg, O_2 sat. 89%. Wheezes still heard in
		all lung fields but not as loud. Wheezing no
		longer audible without stethoscope. Pt. still
		dyspneic but states breathing has eased. Can
		speak several words at a time. Skin still pale,
		use of accessory muscles not as prominent.
		RR 24 and less labored. P 104, BP 138/86. Dr.
		Murdock notified at 1000 of ABG results and
		assessment findings. No new orders. Repeat
		nebulized albuterol treatment ordered and
		given by Mr. Striker. ————— Lesley Neilsen, RN

Status epilepticus

- Status epilepticus is a state of continuous seizure activity or the occurrence of two or more sequential seizures without full recovery of consciousness in between.
- It can result from abrupt withdrawal of anticonvulsant drugs, hypoxic encephalopathy, acute head trauma, metabolic encephalopathy, or septicemia secondary to encephalitis or meningitis.
- Status epilepticus is a life-threatening event that requires immediate treatment to avoid or reduce the risk of brain damage.
- If your patient develops status epilepticus:
  - Notify the practitioner right away.
  - Maintain a patent airway.
  - Protect the patient from harm.
  - Administer anticonvulsant drugs, as ordered.

The write stuff

- Record:
  - date and time that the seizure activity started
  - its duration
  - precipitating factors.
- Note whether the patient reported warning signs (such as an aura).
- Document the characteristics of the seizure and related patient behaviors, such as:
  - pupil characteristics
  - level of consciousness
  - breathing
  - skin color
  - bowel and bladder continence
  - body movements.

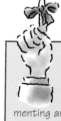

Memory jogger

Here's a TIP for documenting an episode of status epilepticus. Include:

Time and date seizure activity started

Its duration

Precipitating factors.

- Record:
  - practitioner's name
  - time of notification
  - orders received, such as I.V. administration of anticonvulsants.
- Document your actions, such as:
  - maintaining a patent airway
  - suctioning
  - patient positioning
  - loosening of clothing
  - monitoring vital signs
  - neurologic assessment.
- Record the patient's response to treatment and your ongoing assessments.
- Note that you stayed with the patient throughout the seizure.
- Record education and emotional support given to the patient and his family.
- Record your assessment of the patient's postictal status.
- On the appropriate flow sheets, record:
  - frequent assessments
  - vital signs
  - neurologic assessments.

09/17/06	1730	Housekeeper Norma Jennings called for help
		and reported noticing pt. lose consciousness.
		Pt. had full body stiffness, followed by
		alternating episodes of muscle spasm and
		relaxation. Breathing was labored and sonorous.
		Pt. was incontinent of bowel and bladder. Skin
		ashen color. Seizure lasted approx. 2 min.
		Clothing loosened and pt. placed on Ⓛ side. Pt.
		unconscious after seizure, not responding to
		verbal stimuli. Airway patent; pt. breathing on
		own. P 92, BP 128/62, RR 18 and uneven.
		Approx. 1 min later, seizure recurred and was
		continuous. Dr. Palmer notified of assessment
		findings at 1703; diazepam 5 mg I.V. X 1 dose
		ordered and given STAT and phenytoin 1 g
		I.V. X 1 dose ordered and given STAT.
		Started 35% O₂ via facemask. Seizure stopped
		at 1710. Stayed with pt. throughout seizures.
		Pt. breathing on own, RR 20 and regular, O₂
		sat. 95%. P 88 and regular, BP 132/74,
		tympanic T 98.2° F. Pt. sleeping and not
		responding to verbal stimuli. O₂ mask removed.
		Incontinence care provided. Will maintain on
		Ⓛ side and monitor closely during recovery.
		See flow sheets for documentation of
		frequent VS, I/O, and neuro. signs. ————
		———————————— Audrey Horne, RN

Stroke

- A stroke is a sudden impairment of cerebral circulation in one or more of the blood vessels supplying the brain.
- A stroke interrupts or diminishes oxygen supply and commonly causes serious damage or necrosis in brain tissues.
- Clinical features vary with the artery affected and the portion of the brain it supplies, the severity of damage, and the extent of collateral circulation.
- A stroke may be caused by thrombosis, embolus, or intracerebral hemorrhage.
- Stroke may be confirmed by computed tomography (CT) scan or magnetic resonance imaging.
- Treatment options vary, depending on the cause of the stroke.
- The sooner you detect signs and symptoms of a stroke, the sooner the patient can receive treatment and the better his prognosis will be.
- If you suspect a patient is having or has had a stroke:
  - Ensure a patent airway, breathing, and circulation.
  - Perform a neurologic examination.
  - Alert the practitioner of your findings.

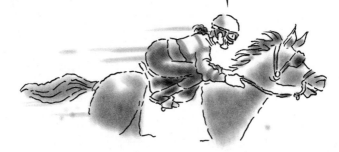

Remember, the faster you detect stroke symptoms, the faster your patient gets treated and the better his prognosis will be!

The write stuff

- Record the date and time of your entry.
- Record the events leading up to the suspected stroke and the signs you noted.
- If the patient can communicate, record symptoms using his own words.
- Document your assessment of the patient's airway, breathing, and circulation and your interventions.
- Document:
  - name of the practitioner notified
  - time of notification
  - whether orders were received.
- Document the time the CT scan was performed and when results were obtained, if ordered.
- Record your neurologic and cardiovascular assessments, actions taken, and the patient's response.
- Use flow sheets to record:
  - frequent assessments
  - frequent vital signs
  - intake and output
  - I.V. therapy
  - laboratory test and arterial blood gas values.
- Document your frequent neurologic assessments, such as the Glasgow Coma Scale or the National Institutes of Health Stroke Scale.
- Record any patient teaching and emotional support given.

11/10/06	2030	When giving pt. her medication at 2015, noted drooping of L eyelid and L side of mouth. Pt. was in bed breathing comfortably with RR 24, P 112, BP 142/72, axillary T 97.2° F. Breath sounds clear. Normal heart sounds. PEARLA, awake and aware of her surroundings, answering yes and no by shaking head, speech slurred with some words inappropriate. Pt. follows simple commands. L hand grasp weaker than R hand grasp. L foot slightly dropped and weaker than R. Glasgow Coma Scale score of 13. See Glasgow Coma Scale flow sheet for frequent assessments. Skin cool, dry. Peripheral pulses palpable. Capillary refill less than 3 sec. Called Dr. Becker at 2020. Stat CT scan ordered. Administered O_2 at 2 L/min by NC. I.V. infusion of NSS at 30 ml/hr started in R forearm with 18G catheter. Continuous pulse oximetry started with O_2 sat. of 96% on 2 L O_2. Dr. Becker in to see pt. at 2025. Pt. being prepared for transfer to ICU. Dr. Becker will notify family of transfer. —— Grace Van Owen, RN

Substance withdrawal

- Substance withdrawal occurs when a person who's addicted to a substance (alcohol or drugs) suddenly stops taking that substance.
- Withdrawal symptoms may include tremors, nausea, insomnia, seizures, and even death.
- If your patient is at risk for substance withdrawal or shows signs of withdrawal:
  - Contact the practitioner immediately.
  - Anticipate a program of detoxification.
  - Anticipate long-term therapy to combat drug dependence.

The write stuff

- Record the date and time of your entry.
- Document the patient's substance abuse and addiction history, noting:
  - substance used
  - amount and frequency of use
  - date and time when last used
  - any history of withdrawal.
- Note specific manifestations that the patient had during previous withdrawals.
- Use a flow sheet that lists the signs and symptoms associated with withdrawal from specific substances.
- Document current blood, urine, and alcohol breath test results.
- Document your frequent assessments of signs and symptoms of withdrawal.
- Document:
  - names of individuals notified regarding the patient (such as the practitioner, substance abuse counselor, social worker)
  - date, time, and reason of notification.

- Document orders or instructions received, your nursing actions, and the patient's response.
- Document any patient education and emotional support given.

| 09/17/06 | 1000 | Pt. admitted to Chemical Dependency Unit for withdrawal from ethanol. Has a 30-year history of alcohol dependence and states, "I can't keep this up anymore. I need to get off the booze." Reports drinking a fifth of vodka per day for the last 2 months and that her last drink was today shortly before admission. Her blood alcohol level is 0.15%. She reports having gone through the withdrawal process four times before but has never completed rehabilitation. Reports the following symptoms during previous withdrawals: anxiety, nausea, vomiting, irritability, and tremulousness. Currently demonstrates no manifestations of ethanol withdrawal. Dr. Katz notified of pt.'s admission and blood alcohol level results. Orders received. Lorazepam 2 mg P.O. given at 0930. Pt. instructed regarding s/s of ethanol withdrawal and associated nursing care. She expressed full understanding of the information. Will reinforce teaching when blood tests reveal no alcohol in blood. ———————————————— Laura Benjamin, RN |

Suicide precautions

- Patients who have been identified as being at risk for self-harm or suicide are placed on some form of suicide precautions based on the gravity of the suicidal intent.
- If your patient has suicidal ideations or makes a suicidal threat, gesture, or attempt:
  - Contact the practitioner immediately and institute suicide precautions.
  - Follow facility policy for a potentially suicidal patient.
  - Notify the nursing supervisor, other members of the health care team, and the risk manager.
  - Update the patient's care plan.

Making a case

Legal responsibilities when caring for a suicidal patient

Whether you work on a psychiatric unit or a medical unit, you'll be held responsible for the decisions you make about a suicidal patient's care. If you're sued because your patient has harmed himself while in your care, the court will judge you on the basis of:
- whether you knew (or should have known) that the patient was likely to harm himself
- whether, knowing he was likely to harm himself, you exercised reasonable care in helping him avoid injury or death.

The write stuff

- Record the date and time that suicide precautions were initiated and the reasons for the precautions.
- Chart:
  - time that you notified the practitioner and other people involved in making this decision
  - names of those notified
  - orders received.
- Document the measures taken to reduce the patient's risk of self-harm, such as:
  - removing potentially dangerous items from the patient's environment
  - accompanying the patient to the bathroom
  - placing the patient in a room with sealed windows that is close to the nurses' station.
- Record the level of observation, such as close or constant observation, and who's performing the observation.
- Document that the patient was instructed about the suicide precautions and his response.
- Maintain a suicide precautions flow sheet that includes:
  - patient's mood, behavior, and location
  - nursing interventions performed
  - patient's response to interventions.

10/17/06	1600	Pt. stated, "Every year about this time, I think about offing myself." History of self-harm 1 year ago when pt. lacerated both wrists on the 3rd anniversary of his father's suicide. States that he has been thinking about cutting his wrists again. Dr. Frost notified and pt. placed on suicide precautions. Julie Chan, RN, nursing supervisor, and Harry Truman, risk manager, also notified. Pt. placed in room closest to nurses' station, verified that the sealed window can't be opened. With pt. present, personal items inventoried and those potentially injurious were placed in the locked patient belongings cabinet. Instructed pt. that he must remain in sight of the assigned staff member at all times, including being accompanied to the bathroom and on walks on the unit. Bobby Briggs is assigned to constantly observe pt. this shift. Pt. contracted for safety, stating, "I won't do anything to hurt myself." See flow sheet for q15min assessments of mood, behavior, and location. ———————————— Earle Windom, RN

Surgical incision care

- In addition to documenting vital signs and level of consciousness when the patient returns from surgery, pay particular attention to maintaining records about the surgical incision and drains and the care that you provide.
- Read the records that travel with the patient from the postanesthesia care unit.
- Look for a practitioner's order indicating who will perform the first dressing change.

The write stuff

- Chart the date, time, and type of wound care performed.
- Describe the wound's:
  - appearance (size, condition of margins, and necrotic tissue, if any)
  - odor (if any)
  - location of any drains
  - drainage characteristics (type, color, consistency, and amount).
- Document the condition of the skin around the incision.
- Record the type of dressing and tape applied.
- Document additional wound care procedures provided, such as:
  - drain management
  - irrigation
  - packing
  - application of a topical medication.
- Record the patient's tolerance of the wound care.

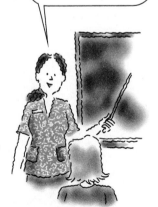

Document your discharge instructions and your patient's understanding of them.

- If you detect abnormalities or have concerns, document:
  - name of the practitioner notified
  - time of notification
  - orders received.
- Note explanations or instructions given to the patient.
- Record wound care instructions and pain management measures on the nursing care plan.
- Document the color and amount of measurable drainage on an intake and output form.
- Document discharge teaching and the patient's understanding of instructions.

12/10/06	0830	Dressing removed from 8-cm midline
		abdominal incision; no drainage noted on
		dressing. Incision well-approximated and
		intact with staples. Margin ecchymotic. Skin
		around incision without redness, warmth, or
		irritation. Small amt. of serosanguineous
		drainage cleaned from lower end of incision
		with NSS and blotted dry with sterile gauze. 3
		dry sterile 4" X 4" gauze pads applied and held
		in place with paper tape. Jackson Pratt drain
		intact in LLQ draining serosanguineous fluid,
		emptied 40 ml. See I/O sheet for drainage
		records. Jackson Pratt insertion site without
		redness or drainage. Split 4" X 4" gauze
		applied around Jackson Pratt drain and taped
		with paper tape. Pt. stated he had only minor
		discomfort before and after the dressing
		change and that he didn't need any pain meds.
		Pt. instructed to call nurse if dressing
		becomes loose or soiled and for incision pain.
		Pt. demonstrated how to splint incision with
		pillow during C&DB exercises. ————————
		———————————— Abby Perkins, RN

Surgical site identification

- To prevent wrong-site surgery and improve the overall safety of patients undergoing surgery, the Joint Commission on Accreditation of Healthcare Organizations launched the Universal Protocol for Preventing Wrong Site, Wrong Procedure, Wrong Person Surgery in 2004.
- This protocol encompasses three important steps:
  - *Preoperative verification process*, which ascertains that all relevant documents, images, and tests are on hand and have been evaluated before surgery; any inconsistencies must be resolved before starting surgery. Two patient identifiers should be used to verify the patient's identity throughout the process.
  - *Marking of the operative site* by the surgeon performing the surgery, with the involvement of the awake and aware patient, if possible. The mark should be the surgeon's initials or the word "yes" at or near the incision site.

  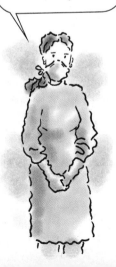

  > Taking a "time out" before surgery is an important step in assuring patient safety.

  - A "time out" immediately before surgery is started, in the location where the surgery is to be performed, so that the entire surgical team can confirm the correct patient, surgical procedure, surgical site, patient position, and any implants or special equipment requirements.
- Most facilities use a detailed checklist to make sure that all steps of the verification process have been completed.

- Each member of the team should document the checks that they performed to ensure proper surgical site identification.

The write stuff

- Document the date, time, and your initials in the area of the checklist that you completed.
- Sign your full name and initials in the signature space provided when using initials on a checklist.
- Record any discrepancies in the verification process on the checklist with a description of actions taken to rectify the discrepancy.
- Include the names of any people notified and their actions.
- Document preoperatively that:
  – you identified the patient using two identifiers
  – the patient understands the procedure and can correctly describe the surgery and identify the surgical site
  – the consent form has been signed and includes the name of the surgery and the surgical site
  – the medical record was checked for the physical examination, medication record, laboratory studies, radiology and electrocardiogram reports, and anesthesia and surgical records and that the medical record is consistent with the type of surgery planned and the identified surgical site.
- Document intraoperatively that:
  – the patient was identified by staff using two identifiers
  – the surgical procedure was confirmed by the staff
  – the surgical site is marked and the patient or family member verified that the marked surgical site was correct
  – the medical record is consistent with the planned surgery and surgical site
  – the availability of implants and special equipment, if relevant, was confirmed.

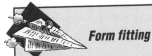

Form fitting

Preoperative surgical identification checklist

A preoperative surgical identification checklist, such as the one below, is commonly used to ensure the safety of patients undergoing surgery.

PREOPERATIVE SURGICAL IDENTIFICATION CHECKLIST

Patient's name _Charlie Kauffman_ Date _01/06/07_ Time _1032_
Medical record number _123456_ Initials _NC_

Preoperative verification	Health team member initials	Date	Time
Patient identified using two identifiers	NC	01/06/07	1032
Informed consent with surgical procedure and site (side/level) signed and in chart	NC	01/06/07	1045
History and physical complete and in chart	NC	01/06/07	1045
Laboratory studies reviewed and in chart	NC	01/06/07	1045
Radiology and ECG reports reviewed and in chart	NC	01/06/07	1045
Medications listed in chart	NC	01/06/07	1045
Patient/family member/guardian verbalizes surgical procedure and points to surgical site	NC	01/06/07	1055
Surgical site marked	AD	01/06/07	1100
Patient, surgery, and marked site verified by patient/family/guardian	NC	01/06/07	1100
Surgical procedure and site, medical record, and tests consistent	NC	01/06/07	1100
Proper equipment and implants available	NC	01/06/07	1100
Describe any discrepancies and actions taken:	N/A		

Preoperative surgical identification checklist *(continued)*

"Time out" verification	Health team member initials	Date	Time
Patient verification with two identifiers	BT	01/06/07	1135
Surgical site verified	BT	01/06/07	1135
Surgical procedure verified	BT	01/06/07	1135
Implants and equipment available	N/A		
Verbal verification of team obtained	BT	01/06/07	1135
Describe any discrepancies and actions taken:	N/A		

Signature *Nancy Cage, RN*   Initials _NC_
Signature *Howard Dunn, RN*   Initials _HD_
Signature *Beverly Thomas, RN*   Initials _BT_

- In the operating room, before the surgical procedure starts, document that a "time out" occurred after a final verification, which should include:
  - verbal consensus by the entire surgical team of identification of the correct patient, surgical site, and surgical procedure and the availability of implants and special equipment, if needed
  - any discrepancy in verification during the "time out" and interventions taken to correct the discrepancy.

Suture removal

- The goal of suture removal is to remove skin sutures from a healed wound without damaging newly formed tissue.
- The timing of suture removal depends on:
  - shape, size, and location of the sutured incision
  - absence of inflammation, drainage, and infection
  - patient's general condition.
- Usually, for a sufficiently healed wound, sutures are removed 7 to 10 days after they're inserted.
- Techniques for removal depend on the method of suturing; however, all techniques require sterile procedure to prevent contamination.
- Although sutures are usually removed by a practitioner, a nurse may remove them in some facilities on the practitioner's order.

The write stuff

- Record the date and time of suture removal.
- Note that you explained the procedure to the patient.
- Include:
  - type and number of sutures
  - appearance of the suture line
  - whether a dressing or butterfly strips were applied.

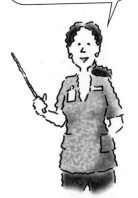

Be sure to define the line. Describe the appearance of the suture line in your documentation.

- Document signs of wound complications as well as:
  - name of the practitioner that you notified
  - time of notification
  - orders received.
- Record the patient's tolerance of the procedure.
- Document patient education given.

| 12/14/06 | 1030 | Order written by Dr. Fleischman for nurse to remove sutures from Ⓛ index finger. Suture line well-approximated and healed. Site clean and dry, no redness or drainage noted. Procedure for suture removal explained to pt. All three sutures removed without difficulty. Dry bandage applied to finger, according to dr.'s order. Pt. didn't c/o pain or discomfort after removal. Explained incision care to pt. and gave written instructions. Pt. verbalized understanding of instructions. ————————— *Maggie O'Connell, RN* |

T

Telephone order

- Ideally, you should accept only written orders from a practitioner.
- Telephone orders are acceptable to expedite care when:
  - a patient needs immediate treatment and the practitioner isn't available to write an order
  - new information, such as laboratory data, is available that doesn't require a physical examination.
- Telephone orders are for the patient's well-being, not strictly for convenience.
- They should be given directly to you, rather than through a third party.
- Carefully follow facility policy and regulating standards on accepting and documenting a telephone order.
- When you receive a telephone order:
  - write it down immediately
  - read it back to the person who gave you the order for verification.
- Make sure the practitioner countersigns the order within the set time limits.
- Without the practitioner's signature, you may be held liable for practicing medicine without a license.

The write stuff

- Note the date and time.
- Record the telephone order verbatim on the practitioner's order sheet while the practitioner is still on the telephone.

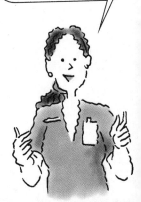

Call it common sense. When you get a telephone order, write it down and read it back.

- Note that you read the order back and received confirmation that it's correct.
- Write "T.O." for telephone order; don't use "P.O." for phone order; that abbreviation could be misinterpreted to mean "by mouth."
- Write the practitioner's name and sign your name.
- If another nurse listened to the order with you, have her sign the order as well.
- Draw lines through any blank spaces in the order.

12/04/06	0900	Demerol 75 mg and Vistaril 50 mg I.M. now
		for pain. Order read back to Dr. Nance, who
		confirmed it. ————————
		———————— T.O. Dr. Nance/Ellen Warren, RN

Thrombolytic therapy

- Thrombolytic drugs, such as alteplase, reteplase, anistreplase, and streptokinase, are used to dissolve a preexisting clot or thrombus, commonly in an acute or emergency situation.
- They're used to treat acute myocardial infarction, pulmonary embolism, acute ischemic stroke, deep vein thrombosis, arterial thrombosis, and arterial embolism and to clear occluded arteriovenous and I.V. cannulas.
- Patients receiving these drugs must be closely monitored for bleeding and allergic reactions.

The write stuff

- Record the date and time of your note.
- Chart the name, dosage, frequency, route, and intended purpose of the thrombolytic drug.
- Note whether the desired response is observed, such as:
  - cessation of chest pain
  - return of electrocardiogram changes to baseline
  - clearing of a catheter
  - improved blood flow to a limb.
- Document your cardiopulmonary, renal, and neurologic assessments.
- Chart vital signs frequently, according to facility policy.
- Record partial thromboplastin time and other coagulation studies.
- Document your frequent assessments of signs and symptoms of complications, such as bleeding, allergic reaction, or hypotension.
- If you observe complications or abnormal laboratory test values, note:
  - name of the practitioner notified and time of notification
  - orders received
  - your interventions
  - patient's response to interventions.

- Document other nursing interventions related to thrombolytic therapy, such as measures to avoid trauma.
- Use flow sheets to record:
  - frequent assessments
  - vital signs
  - hemodynamic measurements
  - intake and output
  - I.V. therapy
  - laboratory test values.
- Include patient teaching and emotional care provided.

09/18/06	1010	Pt. receiving streptokinase 100,000 International Units/hr by I.V. infusion for Ⓛ femoral artery thrombosis. Ⓛ leg and foot cool, dorsalis pedis pulse now faintly palpable, 2 sec capillary refill in Ⓛ foot, able to wiggle Ⓛ toes. P 82 and regular, BP 138/72, RR 18 unlabored, oral T 97.2° F. Breath sounds clear, no dyspnea. Normal heart sounds, skin warm and pink (except for Ⓛ leg), no edema. Alert and oriented to time, place, and person. No c/o headache, hand grasps strong and equally bilaterally, PERRLA. Speech clear and coherent. Voiding on own, urine output remains greater than 75 ml/hour. Urine and stool negative for blood, no flank pain. No bruising, bleeding, or hematomas noted. No c/o itching, nausea, chills. No rash noted. Maintaining pt. on bed rest. Avoiding I.M. injections. See flow sheets for documentation of frequent assessments, VS, I/O, and lab values. Reinforced the purpose of thrombolytic therapy in dissolving clot and the need to observe for bleeding. Pt. verbalized understanding that he's to report blood in urine or stool, headache, and flank pain. —————————————————————— Damon Bradley, R.N.

Tracheostomy care

- Tracheostomy care is performed to:
  - ensure airway patency of the tracheostomy tube by keeping it free from mucus buildup
  - maintain mucous membrane and skin integrity
  - prevent infection
  - provide psychological support.
- The patient may have one of three types of tracheostomy tubes: uncuffed, cuffed, or fenestrated.
- An uncuffed tracheostomy tube:
  - may be plastic or metal
  - allows air to flow freely around the tube and through the larynx, reducing the risk of tracheal damage.
- A cuffed tube:
  - is made of plastic
  - is disposable
  - doesn't require periodic deflating to lower pressures
  - reduces the risk of tracheal damage.
- A fenestrated tube:
  - is made of plastic
  - permits speech through the upper airway when the external opening is capped and the cuff is deflated
  - allows easy removal of the inner cannula for cleaning.
- When using any one of these tubes, use sterile technique to prevent infection until the stoma has healed.
- When caring for a recently performed tracheotomy, use sterile gloves at all times.
- After the stoma has healed, clean gloves may be used.

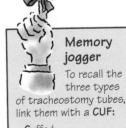

Memory jogger

To recall the three types of tracheostomy tubes, link them with a **CUF**:

Cuffed

Uncuffed

Fenestrated.

The write stuff

- Record the date and time of tracheostomy care.
- Document the type of care performed.
- Describe the amount, color, consistency, and odor of secretions.
- Chart the condition of the stoma and the surrounding skin.
- Note the patient's respiratory status.
- Record:
  – duration of any cuff deflation
  – amount of any cuff inflation
  – cuff pressure readings and specific body position.
- If complications occur, note:
  – name of the practitioner notified
  – time of notification
  – orders received
  – interventions performed
  – patient's response to interventions.
- Document the patient's tolerance of the procedure.
- Include patient education performed.

11/19/06	2200	Trach. care performed using sterile technique. Wiped skin around stoma and outer cannula with sterile gauze soaked in NSS. Dried area with sterile gauze and applied sterile trach. dressing. Skin around stoma intact, no redness. Inner cannula cleaned with hydrogen peroxide and wire brush. Small amount of creamy white, thick, odorless secretions noted. Trach. ties clean and secure. Before procedure, RR 18 and regular, unlabored. Breath sounds clear. After trach. care, RR 16 and regular, with clear breath sounds. Pt. verbalized no discomfort or respiratory distress. Pt.'s wife verbalized desire to assist with procedure when next scheduled to be performed. ———— Jaime Depp, R.N

Tracheostomy suctioning

- Tracheostomy suctioning involves removing secretions from the trachea or bronchi by means of a catheter inserted through the tracheostomy tube.
- Tracheostomy suctioning also stimulates the cough reflex.
- This procedure helps maintain a patent airway to:
  – promote the optimal exchange of oxygen and carbon dioxide
  – prevent pneumonia that results from pooling of secretions.
- Requiring strict sterile technique, tracheostomy suctioning should be performed as frequently as the patient's condition warrants.

The write stuff

- Record the date and time that you performed tracheostomy suctioning as well as the reason for suctioning.
- Document the amount, color, consistency, and odor of the secretions.
- Note any complications as well as nursing actions taken and the patient's response to them.
- Record any pertinent data regarding the patient's response to the procedure.
- Include any patient education given.

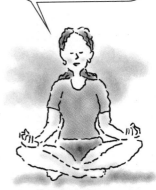

Don't zone out. Remember to perform tracheostomy suctioning as often as necessary.

11/19/06	2145	Pt. coughing but unable to raise secretions.
		Skin dusky. P 98, BP 110/78, RR 30. Breaths
		noisy and labored. Explained suction procedure
		to pt. Using sterile technique, suctioned
		moderate amount of creamy, thick, odorless
		secretions from tracheostomy tube. After
		suctioning, skin pink, respirations quiet, P 88,
		BP 112/74, RR 24. Breath sounds clear. Pt.
		resting comfortably in bed; states he needs to
		cough and deep-breathe more frequently.
		———————————————— Shelly Tambo, RN

Tube feeding

- Tube feeding involves the delivery of a liquid feeding formula directly to the stomach (known as *gastric gavage*), duodenum, or jejunum.
- Tube feeding is typically indicated for a patient who can't eat normally because of dysphagia or oral or esophageal obstruction or injury.
- Tube feedings may also be given to an unconscious or intubated patient or to a patient recovering from GI tract surgery who can't ingest food orally.
- Duodenal or jejunal feedings decrease the risk of aspiration because the formula bypasses the pylorus.
- Jejunal feedings reduce pancreatic stimulation; thus, the patient may require an elemental diet.
- Patients usually receive tube feedings on an intermittent schedule.
- For duodenal or jejunal feedings, most patients tolerate a continuous slow drip.
- Liquid nutrient solutions come in various formulas for administration through a nasogastric tube, small-bore feeding tube, gastrostomy or jejunostomy tube, percutaneous endoscopic gastrostomy or jejunostomy tube, or gastrostomy feeding button.
- Tube feedings are contraindicated in patients who have no bowel sounds or a suspected intestinal obstruction.

The write stuff

- Record the date and time of your entry.
- Document:
  - abdominal assessment findings (including tube exit site, if appropriate)
  - amount of residual gastric contents
  - verification of tube placement
  - amount, type, strength, and time of feeding
  - tube patency.

- Record the patient's tolerance of the feeding, including complications, such as nausea, vomiting, cramping, diarrhea, or abdominal distention.
- Note the result of any laboratory tests, such as urine and serum glucose, serum electrolyte, and blood urea nitrogen levels as well as serum osmolality.
- If complications such as hyperglycemia, glycosuria, and diarrhea occur, document:
  - name of the practitioner notified
  - time of notification
  - orders received
  - interventions performed
  - patient's response to interventions.
- Record the patient's hydration status.
- Note any drugs or treatments to relieve constipation or diarrhea.
- Include the date and time of administration set changes and the results of specimen collections.
- Describe oral and nasal hygiene and dressing changes provided.
- Document patient education given.
- On the intake and output sheet, record:
  - the date
  - volume of formula
  - volume of water.

11/25/06	0700	Full-strength Pulmocare infusing via Flexiflow
		pump through Dobhoff tube in ® nostril at
		50 ml/hr. Tube placement confirmed by
		aspirated gastric contents with pH of 5 and
		grassy-green color. 5 ml residual noted. HOB
		maintained at 45-degree angle. Pt. denies N/V,
		abdominal cramping. Active bowel sounds
		auscultated in all 4 quadrants, no abdominal
		distention noted. Mucous membranes moist,
		no skin tenting when pinched. Nares cleaned
		with cotton-tipped applicator dipped in NSS.
		Water-soluble lubricant applied to nares and
		lips. Skin around nares intact; no redness
		around tape noted. Helped pt. to brush teeth.
		Diphenoxylate elixir 2.5 mg given via tube feed
		for continuous diarrhea. Tube flushed with
		50 ml H_2O q4hr, as ordered. See I/O sheet
		for shift totals. Urine dipstick neg. for
		glucose. Blood drawn this a.m. for serum
		glucose, electrolytes, and osmolality. Instructed
		pt to tell nurse of any discomfort or
		distention. ———————— Michelle Moore, RN

Unlicensed assistive personnel care

- The American Nurses Association defines unlicensed assistive personnel (UAP) as individuals trained to function in an assistive role to the registered professional nurse in the provision of patient care activities, as delegated by and under the supervision of that nurse.
- The nurse should only delegate care that the UAP is competent to perform.
- The nurse must:
  – evaluate the outcome of delegating a task
  – make sure that the task and outcome are accurately documented in the medical record.
- If your facility doesn't allow UAPs to document in the patient record:
  – determine what care was provided
  – assess the patient and the task performed (for example, a dressing change)
  – document your findings.
- If your facility allows UAPs to chart, you may have to countersign their notes.
- If your facility's policy states that the UAP must provide care in your presence, don't countersign unless you actually witness her actions.
- If the policy states that your presence isn't required, your countersignature indicates:
  – the note describes care that the UAP had the authority and competence to perform
  – you verified that the procedure was performed.
- Unless your facility authorizes or requires you to witness someone else's notes, your signature will make you responsible for anything put in the notes above it.

Help desk

Supervising unlicensed assistive personnel

If you supervise unlicensed assistive personnel (UAP), you're responsible and liable for their performance. Limit your liability by educating yourself and advocating that your employer establish policies that clearly delineate the responsibilities of registered nurses, licensed practical nurses, and UAPs. Here are some other tips:

• Attend all educational programs your employer sponsors with respect to supervising UAPs.

• Encourage your supervisors to establish a written policy that defines the actions UAPs may take.

• Work cooperatively with UAPs in your clinical setting. If your employer decides to use UAPs, it's in your patients' best interest to establish a solid working relationship.

• Educate your patients about what UAPs can and can't do for them during your assigned work time. This will help them ask the appropriate individuals to assist them with their needs.

• If problems or disagreements arise over the appropriate functions for UAPs, report to your nursing supervisor for immediate resolution.

• Review your state nurse practice act for provisions regarding delegation to UAPs. Follow all criteria for proper delegation set forth in the act.

• Stay current with your state nursing board's recommendations on the use of UAPs.

The write stuff

- Record the date and time of your entry.
- If UAPs aren't allowed to chart, be sure to record the full name of the UAP who provided care (not just her initials).
- Describe the care that the UAP performed.
- Document your assessment of the patient.

| 12/12/06 | 0930 | Morning care provided by UAP Chris Stevens, who stated that pt. was unsteady on feet walking to bathroom to wash up. Went to see pt., who states that "Ms. Stevens gave me a thorough sponge bath today." Explained to pt. that she was to call for assistance if she needed to get out of the chair. Pt. verbalized understanding. Call bell placed within pt.'s reach. Pt. demonstrated proper use of call bell. ——————— Tammy Hill, R.N |

Urinary catheter (indwelling) insertion

- Also known as a *Foley* or *retention catheter,* an indwelling urinary catheter is inserted into and remains in the bladder to provide continuous urine drainage.
- A balloon inflated at the catheter's distal end prevents it from slipping out of the bladder after insertion.
- Use sterile technique when inserting a urinary catheter.
- Insertion should be performed with extreme care to prevent injury to the patient and possible infection.
- Indications for urinary catheter insertion include:
  - to relieve bladder distention caused by urine retention and allow continuous urine drainage when the urinary meatus is swollen from childbirth, surgery, or local trauma
  - to relieve urine retention caused by urinary tract obstruction due to a tumor or enlarged prostate gland
  - to relieve urine retention from neu-rogenic bladder, paralysis caused by spinal cord injury, or disease
  - to monitor urine output when the patient's illness requires close monitoring.

The write stuff

- Record the date and time that the urinary catheter was inserted.
- Note the size and type of catheter used.
- Describe the amount, color, and other characteristics of the urine emptied from the bladder.

A balloon inflated at a catheter's distal end will keep it from floating up, up, and away.

- Record the intake and output on the patient's intake and output record.
- Describe the patient's tolerance of the procedure.
- Note whether a urine specimen was sent for laboratory analysis.
- Document patient teaching performed.

12/12/06	1115	Explained reason for insertion of indwelling urinary catheter to pt. prior to hysterectomy. Pt. stated she understood the need but wasn't looking forward to its insertion. Reassured her that the insertion shouldn't be painful if she relaxes. Showed her how to do breathing exercises during insertion. #16 Fr. Foley catheter inserted at 1045. Emptied 450 ml from bladder. Urine dark amber, no odor, or sediment. Specimen sent to lab for U/A. Pt. states she has no discomfort and can't feel catheter in place. See I/O flow sheet. ———————————————— Marilyn Roemon, RN

V

Verbal orders

- Errors made interpreting or documenting verbal orders can lead to mistakes in patient care and liability problems for you.
- Verbal orders can be a necessity, especially if you're providing home health care.
- In a health care facility, try to take verbal orders only in an emergency, and according to facility policy, when the practitioner can't immediately attend to the patient.
- You shouldn't accept do-not-resuscitate and no-code orders verbally.
- National patient safety goals expect the person receiving the order to write it down and read it back to the practitioner in its entirety and receive confirmation from the person giving the order.
- Carefully follow facility policy for documenting a verbal order, and use a special form if one exists.
  - Make sure the practitioner countersigns the order within the time limits set by facility policy.
  - Without a countersignature, you may be held liable for practicing medicine without a license.

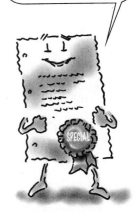

I'm special! Use me or follow your facility's policy to document verbal orders.

The write stuff

- Note the date and time of the order.
- Write the order out verbatim while the practitioner is still present, if possible.
- Document that you read the order back and received verification.
- On the following line, write "V.O." for verbal order, the practitioner's name, and your signature.
- Draw lines through any spaces between the order and your verification of the order.
- Record:
  - type of drug
  - dosage
  - time you administered it
  - any other information your facility's policy requires.

03/23/07	1500	V.O. by Dr. Cusack taken for digoxin 0.125 mg P.O. now and daily in a.m. Furosemide 40 mg P.O. now and daily starting in a.m. Order read back and confirmed. ———————————————— Judith Schilling, RN & ———————————————— Carla Roy, RN ———————————————— James Cusack, MD

Vital signs, frequent

- A patient may require frequent monitoring of vital signs after surgery or certain procedures and diagnostic tests or during a critical illness.
- A frequent vital signs flow sheet allows you to:
  - quickly document vital signs the moment you take them without having to take the time to write a progress note
  - readily detect changes in the patient's condition.
- If recording only vital signs isn't sufficient to give a complete picture of the patient's status, you'll also need to write a progress note.
- Make sure the data on the vital signs flow sheet are consistent with the data in your progress note.

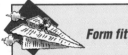

Form fitting

Frequent vital signs flow sheet

When the patient requires frequent vital sign assessments, a flow sheet such as this may help facilitate documentation by eliminating the need to continually make entries in the notation section of the chart. In the example below, blood pressure is monitored every 15 minutes.

FREQUENT VITAL SIGNS FLOW SHEET

Date	Time	Key	BP	P	RR	T	CVP	PAP S/D	PAP M	PAP W
11/13/06	0900	A	122/84	98	18	98⁶				
	0915	A	124/82	94	18					
	0930	A	122/78	92	20					
	0945	A	122/80	94	18					
	1000	A	128/78	94	20					

Signature _Mary Crabtree, RN_   Initials _MC_

Signature _____   Initials _____

The write stuff

- Record the date on the flow sheet.
- Document the specific time each set of vital signs is taken.
- If a significant change in vital signs occurs, write a progress note documenting:
  - details of the change
  - time the practitioner was notified
  - practitioner's name
  - orders received
  - interventions performed
  - patient's response to interventions.

Comments	Titrated I.V.'s	Meds Stat and prn	Initials
			MC
			MC
			MC
			MC
			MC

Key: S = stethoscope   D = Doppler
P = Palpation   T = Transducer
A = Automated

WXYZ

Withholding an ordered medication

- Under certain circumstances, a prescribed medication can't or shouldn't be given as scheduled; for example, you may decide to withhold a stool softener in a patient with diarrhea.
- A patient may be scheduled for a test that requires him to not take a certain medication, or a change in the patient's condition may make the drug inappropriate to give; for example, an antihypertensive medication may have been prescribed for a patient who now has low blood pressure.
- In some circumstances, a patient may refuse a medication; for example, a patient may refuse to take his cholestyramine because he believes it's causing abdominal upset.
- If a medication is withheld, notify the practitioner.

The write stuff
- In your note, document:
  - date and time the medication was withheld
  - reason for withholding the medication
  - name of the practitioner notified and time of notification, if notified
  - practitioner's response, if notified.
- If the practitioner changed a medication order, record and document the new order and the time it was carried out.
- Document any actions taken to safeguard your patient.
- On the medication administration record (MAR):
  - Initial the appropriate box as usual but circle your initials to indicate the medication wasn't given.

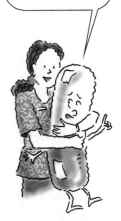

If you withhold me, remember to notify the practitioner.

Form fitting

Withholding an ordered medication

When you withhold an ordered medication, you must document it on the medication administration record. This is usually indicated by circling your initials, as shown below.

Name: _Walt Matthau_   Medical Record #: _123456_

Nurse's full signature, status, and initials
Steve Wonder, RN   _SW_
Theresa Buss, R.N   _TB_

Diagnosis: _Atrial fibrillation_
Allergies: _Sulfa_   Diet: _Cardiac_

Routine/daily orders			Date: 1/24/07		Date: 1/25/07	
Order date	Medications: Dose, route, frequency	Time	Site	Init.	Site	Init.
_1/24/07_ _SW_	_digoxin 0.125 mg I.V. daily_	_0900_	_® subclavian HR-68_	_SW_	_HR-52_	_Ⓣ®_

– Record the correct code indicating why the medication wasn't given, or fill in the appropriate section on the MAR with the date, time, name and dose of the medication withheld, and the reason for withholding the medication.

_01/25/07_	_0900_	_Digoxin 0.125 mg I.V. not given due to pulse_
		less than 60. Dr. Sellers notified that
		medication was withheld. — Theresa Buss, R.N

Wound assessment

- When caring for a patient with a wound, complete a thorough assessment so that you'll have a clear baseline from which to evaluate healing and the appropriateness of therapy.
- Care may need to be altered if the wound doesn't respond to therapy.
- Many facilities have a specific wound care protocol that specifies different treatment plans based on wound assessment.
- A wound should be assessed with each dressing change.
- Many facilities also have a special form or flow sheet on which to document wounds.

The write stuff

- Record the date and time of your entry.
- Include:
  - wound size, including length, width, and depth in centimeters
  - wound shape
  - wound site, drawn on a body plan to document exact location
  - wound stage
  - characteristics of drainage, if any, including amount, color, and presence of odor
  - characteristics of the wound bed, including description of tissue type, such as granulation tissue, slough, or epithelial tissue, and percentage of each tissue type
  - character of the surrounding tissue
  - presence or absence of eschar
  - presence or absence of pain
  - presence or absence of undermining or tunneling (in centimeters).

Form fitting

Wound and skin assessment tool

When performing a wound and skin assessment, pictures can be used to identify the wound site or sites. The sample wound and skin assessment tool below indicates that the patient has a partial-thickness wound, a vascular ulcer, that's red in color on his second toe.

Patient's name _Crockett, James_

Attending physician _Dr. R. Tubbs_

Room number _123-2_   ID number _01726_

WOUND ASSESSMENT

Number	1	2	3	4
Date	12/14/06			
Time	1215			
Location	Ⓛ second toe			
Stage	II			
Appearance	G			
Size (length)	0.5 cm			
Size (width)	1 cm			
Color of floor	RD			
Drainage	O			
Odor	O			
Volume	O			
Inflammation	O			
Size inflam.	O			

KEY:

Stage:
I. Red or discolored
II. Skin break/blister
III. SubQ tissue
IV. Muscle and/or bone

Appearance:
D = Depth
E = Eschar
G = Granulation
IN = Inflammation
NEC = Necrotic
PK = Pink
SL = Slough
TN = Tunneling
UND = Undermining
MX = Mixed (specify)

Color of wound floor:
RD = Red
Y = Yellow
BLK = Black
MX = Mixed (specify)

Drainage:
0 = None
SR = Serous
SS = Serosanguineous
BL = Blood
PR = Purulent

Odor:
0 = None
MLD = Mild
FL = Foul

Volume:
0 = None
SC = Scant
MOD = Moderate
LG = Large

Inflammation:
0 = None
PK = Pink
RD = Red

(continued)

Wound and skin assessment tool (continued)

WOUND ANATOMIC LOCATION
(circle affected area)

Anterior　　　Posterior　　　Left lateral　　　Right lateral

Left foot　　　Right foot　　　Left hand　　　Right hand

Wound care protocol: _Cleaned wound with NSS; dry sterile_
dressing applied.

Signature: _Mark Silver, RN_　　　Date _12/14/06_

12/14/06	1330	Pt. admitted to unit for fem-pop bypass
		tomorrow. Pt. has open wound at tip of
		second Q toe, approx. 0.5 cm X 1 cm X 0.5 cm
		deep. Wound is round with even edges. Wound
		bed is pale with little granulation tissue. No
		drainage, odor, eschar, or tunneling noted. Pt.
		reports pain at wound site; rates pain as 4 on
		scale of 0 to 10, w/10 being the worst pain
		imaginable. Surrounding skin cool to touch,
		pale, and intact. Pt. understands not to cross
		legs or wear tight garments. ————————
		———————————————— Mark Silver, RN

Wound care

- The intent of caring for a surgical wound is to help prevent infection by stopping pathogens from entering the wound.
- Wound care:
  - promotes patient comfort
  - protects the skin surface from maceration and excoriation caused by contact with irritating drainage
  - allows you to measure wound drainage to monitor fluid and electrolyte balance.
- The two principal methods for managing a draining wound are dressing and pouching.
- Dressing is the best choice when skin integrity isn't compromised by caustic or excessive drainage.
- Lightly seeping wounds with drains as well as wounds with minimal purulent drainage can usually be managed with packing and gauze dressings.
- Copious, excoriating drainage calls for pouching to protect the skin.

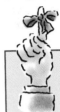

Memory jogger

When providing wound care, remember the three Ps, or purposes, of wound care:

Promotes patient comfort

Protects the skin's surface

Provides the chance to measure wound drainage.

The write stuff

- Document the date and time of the procedure.
- Include the type of wound management used.
- Record the amount of soiled dressing and packing removed.
- Describe:
  - wound appearance (size, condition of margins, and presence of necrotic tissue)
  - odor (if present)
  - type, color, consistency, and amount of drainage for each wound.

- Indicate the presence and location of drains.
- Note additional procedures performed, such as irrigation, packing, or application of a topical medication.
- Record the type and amount of new dressing or pouch applied.
- Note the patient's tolerance of the procedure and any instructions given.
- Document special or detailed wound care instructions and pain management steps on the care plan.
- Record the color and amount of drainage on the intake and output sheet.

11/17/06	1030	Dressing removed from ® mastectomy incision.
		1.5 cm round area of serosanguineous
		drainage noted on dressing. No odor noted.
		11-cm incision well-approximated, staples intact.
		Skin around incision intact, no redness. Site
		cleaned with sterile NSS. Six sterile 4" X 4"
		gauze pads applied. Jackson Pratt drain at
		lateral edge of incision emptied for 10 ml
		serosanguineous fluid, no odor noted. See
		I/O flow sheet for shift totals. Explained
		dressing change and signs and symptoms of
		infection to report. Pt. verbalized
		understanding. Pt. states incision is tender but
		doesn't require pain medication. ———————
		——————————— Michelle Kuzak, RN

Written orders

- No matter who transcribes a practitioner's orders—a registered nurse, licensed practical nurse, or unit secretary—a second person needs to double-check the transcription for accuracy.
- Your unit should also have some method of checking for transcription errors, such as performing 8-hour or 24-hour chart checks.
- When checking a patient's order sheet, always make sure the orders were written for the intended patient.
- Occasionally, an order sheet stamped with one patient's identification plate will inadvertently be placed in another patient's chart.

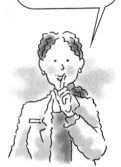

It's no secret that a second person should always double-check a written order for accuracy.

The write stuff

- Night-shift nurses usually:
  - document the 24-hour check by placing a line across the order sheet to indicate that all orders above the line have been checked.
  - sign and date the sheet to verify that they've done the 24-hour medication check.
- The nurse caring for the patient documents the 8-hour check.

01/12/06	1520	Digoxin 0.125 mg P.O. daily Dr. Hanson ——— Mary Bookbinder, RN
01/12/06	1945	Lasix 40 mg I.V. X 1 now. Dr. Hanson ——— Thomas Dolby, RN
01/13/06	0020	24-hour order check. —— Helen Fielding, RN

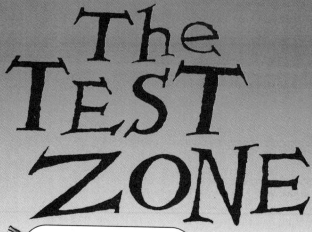

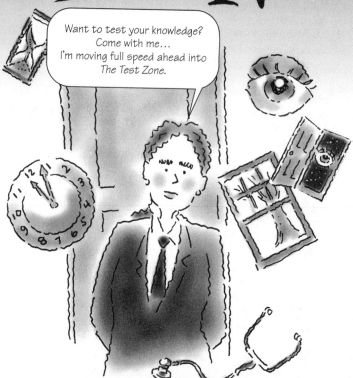

A–C

1. Which action should you take if you suspect that a pediatric patient is being abused?
   A. Continue to observe the child and parent until you are certain abuse has occurred.
   B. Record what you think is happening to the child.
   C. Speak with the parent and child together to gather facts.
   D. Report your suspicions to the appropriate administrator.

2. What would be the most appropriate action to take if your patient decided to leave against medical advice (AMA)?
   A. Tell him that you'll call security if he leaves without being discharged.
   B. Ask him to sit down and review discharge instructions with you before he leaves.
   C. Tell him he must sign an AMA form or you won't let him leave.
   D. Don't accompany him out of the hospital because it was his decision to leave against AMA.

3. Which checks do you need to perform before administering a blood product?
   A. Ask the patient his name and blood type.
   B. Have a family member confirm the patient's name and blood type.
   C. Ask the nursing assistant assigned to the patient to confirm the patient's name and blood type.
   D. Check the patient's identification number and blood type with another licensed health professional.

4. When your patient receives a blood transfusion, what information should be documented on the transfusion record?
   A. Any patient teaching given
   B. The date and time the transfusion was started
   C. The patient's height and weight
   D. The patient's hemoglobin level and hematocrit

5. You have just completed site care for a central venous catheter. Which statement would you use to describe the site in your documentation?

    A. "Site appears benign."

    B. "No redness or drainage noted at site; no tenderness reported."

    C. "No evidence of complications at insertion site."

    D. "Insertion site without signs of infection."

D–H

6. You're caring for a patient who has died from a gunshot wound to the chest. Which action would be most appropriate?

    A. Check to see if the medical examiner will be examining the patient.

    B. Don't allow the family to see the patient because his injuries may be too traumatic for them.

    C. Immediately remove all drains and tubes from the patient to ease the family's distress.

    D. Begin postmortem care immediately so that the family can visit.

7. A patient is receiving epidural analgesia after abdominal surgery. Which assessment parameter would you document to show that the patient isn't experiencing adverse effects?

    A. Respiratory rate of 8 breaths/minute

    B. Blood pressure of 140/80 mm Hg sitting, 90/58 mm Hg standing

    C. Difficulty arousing patient

    D. Patient voiding on his own without difficulty

8. You're performing a risk assessment for falls on a newly admitted patient. Which factor carries the greatest risk of falling?

    A. Taking two or more drugs

    B. Being independent and incontinent

    C. Being confused at times

    D. Having diminished muscle coordination

9. When performing gastric lavage, you should document vital signs:
   A. only if the patient's condition changes.
   B. every 15 minutes until the patient is stable.
   C. when the patient's condition stabilizes.
   D. when the irrigant is instilled.

10. Under the Health Insurance Portability and Accountability Act, you must ensure that your patient's identifiable health information can't be seen by those who aren't involved in his care. Identifiable health information includes:
   A. the patient's room number and health history.
   B. the unit the patient is on and his bed number.
   C. the patient's Social Security number and birth date.
   D. the patient's room number.

I–N

11. Despite preventive measures, a patient falls. Which note would be appropriate to include in the documentation of the incident?
   A. "Patient must have been trying to reach for his phone when he fell out of bed."
   B. "Found patient lying on the floor on his left side, between his bed and bedside table."
   C. "Better staffing could have prevented this fall."
   D. "Patient fell because his call bell wasn't answered in a timely manner."

12. Which statement is appropriate to include in documentation for I.V. catheter insertion?
   A. The patient's veins were tortuous, making venipuncture difficult.
   B. Several attempts at venipuncture were made.
   C. The I.V. was started in the patient's left arm.
   D. A 20G, 1/2″ catheter was inserted in the patient's right forearm during the first attempt.

13. After documenting a patient's head-to-toe assessment, you remember that you forgot to include important information. What's the best way to add a late entry?

A. Write small and squeeze the information in the space where it should have been.

B. Add the missing information to the first available line and label it "late entry."

C. Wait until you have to write another note and add the missing information at that time.

D. Chart your note on a new page and place it in the medical record.

14. You're caring for a patient diagnosed with a stroke. When performing a neurologic assessment, the patient spontaneously opens his eyes, obeys commands, and uses inappropriate words. You assign this patient which Glasgow Coma Score?

A. 11

B. 12

C. 13

D. 14

15. After assisting a practitioner with a lumbar puncture at a patient's bedside, be sure to document:

A. only the procedures that you performed.

B. the date and start and completion times of the procedure.

C. only the specimens you collected.

D. discussions among the health team about the characteristics of the cerebrospinal fluid.

O–Q

16. A patient received a one-time dose of furosemide 20 mg I.V. for heart failure. How should the nurse document the patient's response to this drug?
   A. "Patient diuresing well."
   B. "Urinary output increased within 1 hour of furosemide administration."
   C. "Urinary output 200 ml/hour for 3 hours following administration of furosemide."
   D. "Patient responding well to furosemide."

17. You're assessing your patient's risk of pressure ulcer development using the Braden scale. Which item is assessed by this scale?
   A. Sensory perception
   B. Activities of daily living
   C. Comprehension
   D. Visual acuity

18. Which action must be performed if you discard an opioid dose?
   A. Have a second nurse cosign the discarded dose at the end of the shift.
   B. Flush the discarded dose in the toilet and have another nurse cosign that the dose was discarded.
   C. No action is necessary. Witnessing the discard of an opioid isn't necessary when using an automated storage system.
   D. A second nurse must observe you discard the opioid and then cosign your documentation in the appropriate documentation system.

19. How should you respond when a patient requests to see his medical record?

    A. Get his medical record and allow the patient to read it.

    B. Tell the patient that he isn't allowed to view his medical record.

    C. Ask him if he has any particular concerns about his care.

    D. Fill out an incident report documenting the patient's request.

20. You're making a list of your patient's belongings upon admission. One of the items is a ring. What's an appropriate description of the ring?

    A. Two-carat diamond ring with 14-carat gold band

    B. Oval-shaped clear round stone with white metal band

    C. Expensive diamond engagement ring

    D. Round diamond in four-prong, white gold setting

R–Z

21. You're caring for a rape victim. Which example demonstrates adequate documentation of specimen collection?

    A. "Specimens were collected and left in the refrigerator for the authorities."

    B. "Specimens from various parts of the body were collected."

    C. "Pubic hair combing obtained, labeled, and given to Officer James Smith."

    D. "Cultures obtained and sent to laboratory."

22. What's the appropriate action to take when your patient refuses treatment?

    A. Inform him of the risks involved in not receiving care.

    B. Tell him that he'll be discharged from the hospital if he refuses treatment.

    C. Notify him that the treatment will be administered without his consent.

    D. Tell him that a court order is necessary to refuse treatment.

23. Which action is most appropriate when receiving a telephone order from a practitioner?

    A. Write the order verbatim before reading it back to the practitioner.

    B. Write the order on the practitioner's order sheet using "P.O." to indicate that it's a phone order.

    C. Sign the order with the practitioner's signature because he isn't available to sign for himself.

    D. Write the order after you give the drug.

24. Your patient has refused to take a laxative because he says he has had several loose stools. How should you document this refusal?

    A. Put an "X" through the scheduled administration time on the medication administration record (MAR).

    B. Don't document anything because the drug wasn't administered.

    C. Document near the scheduled time on the MAR that the patient has had several loose stools.

    D. Circle your initials for the appropriate time of administration time on the MAR.

25. Which information must be documented in the operating room immediately before a procedure is started?

    A. "Time-out" being taken

    B. Informed consent being signed

    C. Patient confirming that he understands the procedure

    D. Name of the surgeon performing the surgery

Answers

A–C

1. D. Nurses are required by law to report signs of abuse in children. Follow your facility's policy to report your suspicions to the appropriate administrator.

2. B. Even though your patient is leaving AMA, you need to provide him with routine discharge care. His rights to discharge planning and care are the same as those of a patient's who has been discharged by his practitioner.

3. D. Before administering a blood transfusion, you must document that two licensed health care professionals at the patient's bedside matched the label on the blood bag to the patient's name band and identification number and to the transfusion slip attached to the blood bag for blood group or type, Rh factor, crossmatch data, and blood bank identification number.

4. B. The date and time the transfusion was started and completed should be recorded on the transfusion record.

5. B. Objectively describe the appearance of the central venous catheter insertion site, noting redness, drainage, or tenderness. If drainage is present, describe its appearance.

D–H

6. A. When a patient dies violently or under suspicious circumstances, delay postmortem care until you determine whether the medical examiner needs to examine the patient.

7. D. If the patient is able to void, he isn't experiencing urine retention, an adverse reaction to epidural analgesia. Other adverse effects of epidural analgesia include respiratory depression, sedation, orthostatic hypotension, itching, nausea, headache, back soreness, hypotension, and leg weakness and numbness.

8. B. According to the Risk Assessment for Falls form, being independent and incontinent places the patient at greatest risk for falling.

9. B. Vital signs should be taken before the gastric lavage procedure starts and then every 15 minutes until the patient is stable.

10. C. Identifiable health information includes the patient's name, Social Security number, birth date, identification number, admission and discharge dates, and health history.

I–N

11. B. When filling out an incident report, include only factual, objective information. Avoid speculating, making judgments, or offering opinions.

12. D. After starting an I.V., document the gauge and length of the catheter inserted and the anatomic location of the insertion site. Also include the number of attempts at venipuncture, the type and flow rate of the I.V. solution, the name and amount of medication in the solution (if applicable), adverse reactions, and actions taken to correct them.

13. B. When you must add a late entry, add it to the first available line and label it "late entry" to show that it's out of sequence. Document the late entry as soon as you realize you've omitted information.

14. C. The patient would receive a score of 4 for spontaneous eye opening, 6 for obeying commands, and 3 for using inappropriate words, giving him a total score of 13.

15. B. When you assist in a lumbar puncture procedure, record the date and the start and completion times. Other information that you should chart includes the name of the person performing the procedure, the patient's response to the procedure, adverse reactions, the number of tubes of cerebrospinal fluid that were collected, the time they were sent to the laboratory, and the characteristics of the cerebrospinal fluid.

O–Q

16. C. When you give a one-time drug dose, your documentation should include the patient's response to the drug. The patient's response should be described using objective parameters. Avoid using vague terms and subjective statements.

17. A. The Braden scale assesses the risk of pressure ulcer development by rating the patient in the following areas: sensory perception, moisture, activity, mobility, and nutrition.

18. D. Government regulations require that a second nurse watch you discard all or part of an opioid dose and then document that she witnessed this discard.

19. C. If your patient asks to see his medical record, ask him why he wants to see it. For example, determine if he's just being curious or having concerns about his treatment. Then follow your facility's policy for letting a patient review his medical record.

20. B. Be objective when describing a patient's belongings. Describe the item, noting color, approximate size, style, type, serial numbers, and other distinguishing features. Don't assess the item's value or authenticity.

R–Z

21. C. When documenting specimen collection for a rape victim, make sure you include how and where the specimen was obtained. Also document that the specimen was labeled per facility policy and to whom the specimen was given.

22. A. When a competent patient refuses treatment, inform him of the risks involved in his decision, notify his practitioner, and have the patient sign a refusal-of-treatment form.

23. A. Record the telephone order verbatim on the doctor's order sheet and read it back to the doctor for confirmation. Use "T.O." in your documentation to indicate that it is a telephone order.

24. D. If you withhold a medication, initial the appropriate box on the MAR as usual, but circle your initials to indicate that the drug wasn't given. Document why the drug was withheld in the notes section of the MAR or in your progress notes.

25. A. Documentation of "time-out" must occur in the operating room before a surgical procedure starts and includes verbal consensus by the entire surgical team of patient identity, surgical site and procedure, and special supply availability.

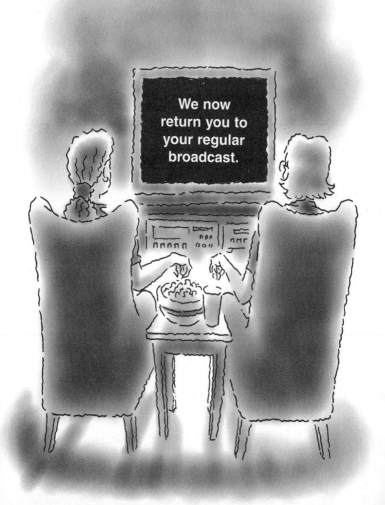

JCAHO National Patient Safety Goals

• The 2007 standards for accreditation of hospitals developed by the Joint Commission on Accreditation of Healthcare Organizations (JCAHO) include the identification of goals, functions, and standards for provision of patient care.

• The purpose of JCAHO's National Patient Safety Goals is to promote improvements in patient safety.

• The goals highlight problematic areas in health care and describe evidence- and expert-based solutions to these problems.

• Because JCAHO recognized that sound system design is intrinsic to the delivery of safe, high-quality health care, the goals focus on system-wide solutions wherever possible.

Summary of the 2007 National Patient Safety Goals

• Improve the accuracy of patient identification.

– Use at least two patient identifiers (don't use patient location) when giving medications or blood products, taking laboratory samples and other specimens for clinical testing, or providing other treatments or procedures.

– Immediately before the start of an invasive procedure, conduct a final verification process to confirm the correct patient, procedure, site, and presence of appropriate documents.

– Re-establish the patient's identity if the practitioner leaves the patient's location before starting the procedure.

– Mark the site unless the practitioner is in continuous attendance from the time of the decision to do the procedure and patient consent to the time of the procedure.

• Improve the effectiveness of communication among caregivers.

– For verbal or telephone orders, or for telephone reporting of critical test results, verify the complete order or test by having the person receiving the information, when possible, write the information down and then read back the complete order or test result in its entirety and receive confirmation.

– Use only approved abbreviations, acronyms, and symbols. A standardized list of abbreviations, acronyms, and symbols that aren't to be used throughout your facility will at minimum consist of JCAHO's do-not-use list and must include three others identified by the facility. JCAHO has developed a list of items to be considered for addition to the "minimum required list" when your facility is expanding its list.

Abbreviations to avoid

To reduce the risk of medical errors, the Joint Commission on Accreditation of Healthcare Organizations (JCAHO) has created an official "Do Not Use" list of abbreviations. In addition, JCAHO offers suggestions for other abbreviations and symbols to avoid.

Official "Do Not Use" List[1]

Do not use	Potential problem	Use instead
U (unit)	Mistaken for "0" (zero), the number "4" (four) or "cc"	Write "unit"
IU (International Unit)	Mistaken for IV (intravenous) or the number 10 (ten)	Write "International Unit"
Q.D., QD, q.d., qd (daily)	Mistaken for each other	Write "daily"
Q.O.D., QOD, q.o.d., qod (every other day)	Period after the Q mistaken for "I" and the "O" mistaken for "I"	Write "every other day"
Trailing zero (X.0 mg)* Lack of leading zero (.X mg)	Decimal point is missed	Write X mg Write 0.X mg

(continued)

Abbreviations to avoid *(continued)*

Do not use	Potential problem	Use instead
MS	Can mean morphine sulfate or magnesium sulfate	Write "morphine sulfate" Write "magnesium sulfate"
MSO_4 and $MgSO_4$	Confused for one another	

1 Applies to all orders and all medication-related documentation that is handwritten (including free-text computer entry) or on pre-printed forms.

* Exception: A "trailing zero" may be used only where required to demonstrate the level of precision of the value being reported, such as for laboratory results, imaging studies that report size of lesions, or catheter/tube sizes. It may not be used in medication orders or other medication-related documentation.

Additional Abbreviations, Acronyms, and Symbols
(For <u>possible</u> future inclusion in the Official "Do Not Use" List)

Do not use	Potential problem	Use instead
> (greater than) < (less than)	Misinterpreted as the number "7" (seven) or the letter "L" Confused for one another	Write "greater than" Write "less than"
Abbreviations for drug names	Misinterpreted due to similar abbreviations for multiple drugs	Write drug names in full

Abbreviations to avoid *(continued)*

Do not use	Potential problem	Use instead
Apothecary units	Unfamiliar to many practitioners Confused with metric units	Use metric units
@	Mistaken for the number "2" (two)	Write "at"
cc	Mistaken for U (units) when poorly written	Write "ml" or "milliliters"
µg	Mistaken for mg (milligrams) resulting in one thousand-fold overdose	Write "mcg" or "micrograms"

– Measure, assess and, if appropriate, take action to improve the timeliness of reporting and the receipt of critical test results and values by the responsible licensed caregiver.

– Your facility will determine critical test results and values that require urgent response and acceptable turnaround times for reporting of these critical test results. These usually include all laboratory and imaging test results reported verbally or by telephone. All results defined as critical by the facility are reported to a responsible licensed caregiver within time frames established by the facility. The "readback" requirement will also apply to critical test results. Documentation should include who you received the critical result from, or who you reported it to, and the date and time.

– If the patient's responsible licensed caregiver isn't available within the time frames, report the critical information to an alternative responsible caregiver.

– Implement a standardized approach to "hand off" communica-

tions, including a chance to ask and respond to questions. Give a complete, safe, hand off communication to the staff member taking over for you. This includes, but isn't limited to, nursing shift changes, temporary responsibility for staff leaving the unit for a short time, anesthesiologists reporting to the postanesthesia care unit nurse, and nursing and doctor hand off from the emergency department to inpatient units, different facilities, nursing homes, and home health care.

- Improve the safety of using medications.
  - Standardize and limit the number of drug concentrations available within the facility.
  - Identify and annually review a list of look-alike and sound-alike drugs used in the facility and take action to prevent errors by the interchange of these drugs.
  - A facility must include on its own list a minimum of 10 look-alike or sound-alike drug combinations from the table JCAHO has issued.
  - Don't store look-alike and sound-alike drugs next to each other.
  - Label all medications, medication containers (syringes, medicine cups, basins), or other solutions on and off the sterile field in perioperative and other procedural settings.
- Eliminate wrong site, wrong patient, wrong procedure surgery.
  - Use an ongoing process of information gathering and verification through all settings.
  - Use a preoperative verification process, such as a checklist, to confirm that the needed documents are present and that all interventions to prepare the patient have been completed.
  - Use a process to mark the surgical site, involve the patient in the marking process, and complete necessary documentation.
  - Perform a "time out" immediately before the procedure starts to verify the patient's identity, correct side and site of the procedure, correct patient position, procedure being performed, and availability of special equipment or implants needed for the procedure.
- Improve the effectiveness of clinical alarm systems.
  - Initiate regular preventive maintenance and testing of alarm systems.
  - Make sure that alarms are activated with appropriate settings and are sufficiently audible with respect to distances and competing noise within the unit.
- Reduce the risk of health care–associated infections.
  - Comply with the Centers for Disease Control and Prevention hand hygiene guidelines. Hand hygiene before entering and after leaving a patient's room and no artificial or long nails are included in these guidelines.

– Manage as sentinel events cases of unanticipated death or major permanent loss of function associated with a health care–associated infection.

• Accurately and completely reconcile medications across the continuum of care.

– Implement a process for obtaining and documenting a complete list of the patient's current medications on admission with the involvement of the patient. This includes a comparison of the medications that the facility provides to those on the list.

– A complete list of the patient's medications is communicated to the next provider of service when a patient is referred or transferred to another setting, practitioner, or level of care within or outside the facility. The complete list should also be given to the patient when he's discharged from the facility.

• Reduce the risk of patient harm resulting from falls.

– Implement a falls risk assessment and falls reduction program and evaluate its effectiveness.

• Reduce the risk of influenza and pneumococcal disease in older adults.

– Develop and implement a protocol for administration and documentation of the flu vaccine.

– Develop and implement a protocol for administration and documentation of the pneumococcus vaccine.

– Develop and implement a protocol to identify new cases of influenza and manage an outbreak.

• Reduce the risk of surgical fires.

– Educate staff, including licensed independent practitioners and anesthesia providers, on how to control heat sources and manage fuels, and establish guidelines to minimize oxygen concentration under drapes.

• Implement applicable National Patient Safety Goals and requirements for components and practitioner sites.

– Inform staff and encourage implementation of the National Patient Safety Goals.

• Encourage active involvement of patients and families in the patient's care as a patient safety strategy.

– Define and communicate methods for patients and families to report concerns about safety and encourage them to do so.

• Prevent health care–associated pressure ulcers.

– Assess and periodically reassess each patient's risk of developing a pressure ulcer and address identified risks.

• Identify safety risks inherent in the facility's patient population.

– Identify patients at risk for suicide.

Electronic health record

- Electronic health record information systems have become one of the strongest trends in documentation. Computerization of medical information can increase efficiency and accuracy in all phases of the nursing process and can help nurses meet the standards set by the American Nurses Association and the Joint Commission on Accreditation of Healthcare Organizations (JCAHO).
- Current computerized systems not only collect, transmit, and organize the information but also suggest nursing diagnoses and provide standardized patient status and nursing interventions, which can be used for care plans and progress notes.
- Computerized systems may even interact with you, prompting you with questions and suggestions about the information that you enter.
- Computers can also be used to help with other types of paperwork, such as nurse management reports, patient classification data, and staffing projections.
- In addition, computers can help identify patient education needs and provide teaching aids and printed information for patients
- Computers can supply data for nursing research and education.

Nursing process

Depending on your facility's software, you might use computers for these nursing processes:

- Assessment: Admission data can be collected via computer terminals. After entering patient data, such as health status, history, chief complaint, and other assessment data, the computer system can flag an entry if data are outside the acceptable range.
- Nursing diagnosis: Most current programs list standard diagnoses with associated signs and symptoms and can suggest one for your patient. However, you still need to use clinical judgment to determine if the suggested diagnosis is right for your patient.
- Planning: To help nurses begin writing a care plan, computer programs can display recommended expected outcomes and interventions for the selected diagnoses. You may also use a computer program to compare and track patient outcomes for a selected group of patients.
- Implementation: Use the computer to record actual interventions and patient-processing information, such as discharge or transfer instructions. Progress notes, medication administration, vital signs, and treatments can also be documented with the computer.

• Evaluation: Use the computer to record evaluation and reevaluation as well as your patient's response to nursing care.

Nursing Minimum Data Set

• The Nursing Minimum Data Set (NMDS) program attempts to standardize nursing information.
• NMDS contains three categories: nursing care, patient demographics, and service elements.
• NMDS allows you to collect nursing diagnosis and intervention data and identify the nursing needs of various patient populations.
• NMDS also lets you track patient outcomes.
• This system helps establish accurate estimates for nursing service costs and provides data about nursing care that may influence health care policy and decision making.
• With the NMDS, you can compare nursing trends locally, regionally, and nationally using data from various clinical settings, patient populations, and geographic areas.
• By comparing trends, you can set realistic outcomes for an individual patient as well as formulate accurate nursing diagnoses and plan interventions.

Nursing outcomes classification

• The Nursing Outcomes Classification (NOC) system provides the first comprehensive standardized method of measuring nursing-sensitive patient outcomes.
• NOC has major implications for nursing administrative practice and the patient care delivery system.
• This system allows the nurse to compare her patients' outcomes to the outcomes of larger groups, according to such parameters as age, diagnosis, and health care setting.

Maintaining confidentiality

• Use of electronic health records have raised issues about the confidentiality of patient information.
• Electronic health records have made patient information more readily accessible to all members of the health care team with access to the computer.
• Nurses need to take measures to ensure the privacy and confidentiality of patient information when using electronic health records.
• When using a computer, make sure the screen is turned so that visitors and other unauthorized people can't see the monitor.
• Change your password frequently and never give your password to another person.

- Choose a password that can't be easily determined by others, such as the name of a pet or child.
- Delete the password of health care workers who are no longer employed at the facility.
- Be sure to log off the computer when you are finished using it.
- Plan and participate in ongoing training sessions regarding confidentiality issues when using electronic health records.
- Be aware that only the nurse caring for the patient should access the patient's medical record.
- Be aware that using an electronic record leaves a trail that can show information that you accessed.
- When using voice-activated systems, make sure visitors and other unauthorized people can't hear your communications.
- Before leaving work, discard computer-generated worksheets, laboratory data, order sheets, and other printouts with patient information in special containers for shredding.

Computer accessibility

- In addition to having a mainframe computer, most health care facilities place personal computers or terminals at workstations throughout the facility so that departmental staff can quickly access vital information.

- Some facilities put terminals at patients' bedsides, making data even more accessible.
- Depending on which type of computer and software your facility has, you may access information by using a keyboard, a light pen, a touch-sensitive screen, a mouse, or your voice.

Voice-activated systems

- A microphone connected to the computer transfers speech into written word.
- Voice-activated systems are most useful in hospital departments that have a high volume of structured reports, such as the operating room.
- Software programs use a specialized knowledge base, nursing words, phrases, and report forms in combination with automated speech recognition (ASR) technology.
- The ASR system requires little or no keyboard use and allows the user to record prompt and complete nursing notes by voice while speaking into a telephone handset.
- The system displays the text on the computer screen.
- These systems increase the speed of reporting and free the nurse from paperwork.
- Noise levels may increase with voice-activated systems and privacy may be compromised if dictation is overheard by others.

E-mail

- E-mail is a convenient form of communication that's fast and always legible.
- E-mail messages between health care providers and between health care providers and patients should be considered part of the patient's medical record.
- The sender of an e-mail message doesn't have to wait in queue, as can happen when using a telephone or fax.
- E-mail leaves a trail of the date and time a message was sent, who sent the message, when the message was received and read, and whether copies were sent to other people.
- Although e-mail messages can be deleted, they can be retrieved through the use of special technology.
- E-mail messages are easy to store and retrieve, if needed.
- A disadvantage of e-mail is that it can be intercepted or forwarded to unintended people.
- E-mail can contain viruses that can unintentionally be sent to other computers.
- E-mail shouldn't be used to transmit urgent messages concerning a patient's health care or critical test results.
- Highly confidential information shouldn't be sent by e-mail.
- Deleting an e-mail can be considered falsification of a patient's medical record.

Advantages of computerized charting

Increases efficiency

- Makes storing and retrieving information fast and easy
- Allows efficient and constant updating of information
- Helps link diverse sources of patient information
- Can quickly and efficiently send request slips and patient information from one terminal to another, which helps ensure confidentiality
- Allows more than one person to view information on a patient at the same time
- May be viewed by providers at different locations—for example, a doctor can enter orders from his office for a patient in the hospital
- Can make online policy and procedure manuals, laboratory manuals, medication information, and other useful information more accessible to nurses
- Saves time and facilitates care by using standardized online orders for certain diagnoses
- Can display information in many ways—for example, laboratory results can be displayed by date or by trends over time

Improves quality of patient care
- Stores data on patient populations
- Facilitates individualized patient assessments
- Supports the use of the nursing process
- Follows facility and JCAHO standards
- Allows written instructions, such as discharge instructions or medication sheets, to be printed for patients

Reduces medical errors
- Uses standard terminology, which improves communication among health care disciplines and promotes more accurate comparisons
- Is always legible
- Can incorporate a facility's standards of care, thereby prompting nurses to enter essential information and take action, such as alerting the nurse that a patient needs a wound care consult or that drug levels need to be drawn when administering certain drugs
- May allow nurses to print out worksheets that detail the treatment and medications a patient requires for the shift
- Uses barcoding of medications, the patient's identification band, and the medication record
- Makes tampering with the health record difficult because changes in the record can be tracked

Disadvantages of computerized charting

Privacy, security, and confidentiality
- Can threaten patient confidentiality if security measures are neglected
- May cause important information to be omitted if software categorizes patient data
- May allow confidential information to be distributed or seen by unauthorized people

Operational issues
- If used incorrectly, may scramble patient information
- Can make information inaccurate or incomplete if limited to standardized phrases
- May be intimidating to workers, especially those who lack typing skills or computer literacy
- May increase errors among people who lack computer literacy
- Makes information temporarily unavailable when the system is down
- Can take extra time if too many nurses try to chart on too few terminals
- Is expensive
- Leaves patient data vulnerable to loss by computer viruses

Selected references

Austin, S. "Ladies and Gentlemen of the Jury, I Present…Nursing Documentation," *Nursing2006* 36(1):56-62, January 2006.

Birmingham, J. "Documentation: A Guide for Case Managers," *Lippincott's Case Management* 9(3):155-57, May-June 2004.

Brous, E.A. "7 Tips on Avoiding Malpractice Claims: Careful Practice and Documentation Help Keep You Out of Court," *TravelNursing2004* 34(6):16-18, June 2004.

Chart Smart: The A-to-Z Guide to Better Nursing Documentation, 2nd ed. Philadelphia: Lippincott Williams & Wilkins, 2007.

Childers, K.P. "Paying a Price for Poor Documentation," *Nursing 2005* 35(11):32hn4-6, November 2005.

Cowden, S., and Johnson, L.C. "A Process for Consolidation of Redundant Documentation Forms," *CIN: Computers, Informatics, Nursing* 22(2):90-93, March-April 2004.

Devine, R. "Issues of Documentation," *Lippincott's Case Management* 9(1):52-53, January-February 2004.

Erlen, J.A. "HIPAA: Clinical and Ethical Considerations for Nurses," *Orthopaedic Nursing* 23(6):410-13, November-December 2004.

Gallagher, P.M. "Maintain Privacy with Electronic Charting," *Nursing Management* 35(2):16-17, February 2004.

Gunningberg, L., and Ehrenberg, A. "Accuracy and Quality in the Nursing Documentation of Pressure Ulcers: A Comparison of Record Content and Patient Examination," *Journal of Wound, Ostomy, and Continence Nursing* 31(6):328-35, November-December 2004.

Hamilton, A.V., et al. "Applied Technology Rounds Out e-Documentation," *Nursing Management* 35(9):44-47, September 2004.

Huffman, M.H., and Cowan, J.A. "Redefine Care Delivery and Documentation," *Nursing Management* 35(2):34-38, February 2004.

Hyde A., et al. "Modes of Rationality in Nursing Documentation: Biology, Biography, and the 'Voice of Nursing,'" *Nursing Inquiry* 12(2):66-77, June 2005.

Iyer, P., et al. *Medical Legal Aspects of Medical Records.* Tucson, Ariz.: Lawyers & Judges Publishing Company, Inc., 2006.

Kaye, W., et al. "When Minutes Count: The Fallacy of Accurate Time Documentation during In-Hospital Resuscitation," *Resuscitation* 65(3):285-90, June 2005.

Kettenbach, G. *Writing SOAP Notes: With Patient/Client Management Formats*, 3rd ed. Philadelphia: F.A. Davis Co., 2004.

Langowski, C. "The Times They Are a Changing: Effects of Online Nursing Documentation Systems," *Quality Management in Health Care* 14(2):121-25, April-June 2005.

McNabney, M.K., et al. "Nursing Documentation of Telephone Communication with Physicians in Community Nursing Homes," *Journal of the American Medical Directors Association* 5(3):180-85, May-June 2004.

"New JCAHO Documentation Guidelines Required Nationwide," *TravelNursing2004* 34(2):2, February 2004.

Owen, K. "Documentation in Nursing Practice," *Nursing Standard* 19(32):48-49, April 2005.

"Quick Tips: Documentation Essentials," *Advances in Skin & Wound Care* 17(2):55, March 2004.

Smith, K., et al. "Evaluating the Impact of Computerized Clinical Documentation," *CIN: Computers, Informatics, Nursing* 23(3): 132-38, May-June 2005.

Smith, L.S. "When a Colleague Falsifies the Record," *Nursing2005* 35(12):76, December 2005.

Sullivan, G.H. "Does Your Charting Measure Up?" *RN* 67(3):61-65, March 2004.

Turpin, P.G. "Transitioning from Paper to Computerized Documentation," *Gastroenterology Nursing* 28(1):61-62, January-February 2005.

Index

A

Abuse, 2-5
  nurse's role in reporting, 4
  signs of, 3
  types of, 2
Activities of daily living, 6-10
  Katz index for, 6
  Lawton scale for, 7
ADLs. *See* Activities of daily living.
Admission, patient's belongings at,
    242-243
Admission assessment form, 11, 12-14i
Advance directive, 15, 16i, 17
Adverse drug effects, 18-19
  MedWatch form for, 18, 19, 20i
Against medical advice discharge,
    21-24
  reasons for, 21
Airway removal, 106-107
Alternate care facility, patient transfer
    to, 256, 257-258i, 259-260
Anaphylactic shock, 317t
Anaphylaxis, 25-27
Aquathermia pad, 141-142
Arrhythmias, 28-29
Arterial line
  insertion of, 30-31
  removal of, 32
Arterial pressure monitoring, 33-34
  indications for, 33

B

Barthel index, 8-10i
Battery, 299

Blood glucose level
  elevated, 137-138
  low, 143-144
  record of, 246-247i
Blood pressure, low, 145-147
Blood transfusion, 35-37
  identification and crossmatching
      procedures for, 35
Blood transfusion reaction, 38, 39i, 40
  delayed, 86-87
Brain death, 41-42
  cardinal signs of, 41

C

Cardiac monitoring, 43-44
  types of, 43
  uses for, 43
Cardiac tamponade, 45-46
Cardiogenic shock, 317t
Cardiopulmonary arrest and resuscita-
    tion, 47, 48-49i, 49-50
Cardioversion, synchronized, 51-52
Caregiver teaching, 249, 254
Central venous catheter
  insertion of, 53-54
  removal of, 55
  site care for, 56
  uses for, 53
Change in patient condition, 57-58
Chest drainage system. *See* Chest
    tube.
Chest pain, 59-60
Chest percussion, 61
Chest physiotherapy, 61

i refers to an illustration; t refers to a table.

Chest tube
  caring for patient with, 62-63
  insertion of, 64-65
  removal of, 66-67
Child abuse, 2, 3, 4
Code record, 48-49i
Cold application, 68-69
Communicable disease reporting,
      70, 72
Communicating condition changes
      over the phone, 57
Correction to documentation, 73
Coughing and deep-breathing
      exercises, 61
Critical value reporting, 74-75
Cultural needs, 76, 77-80i, 80

D

Death, 82-83
Dehydration, 84-85
Delayed transfusion reaction, 86-87
Diagnostic testing, 88
Dialysis, peritoneal, 267-268
Direct arterial monitoring. *See* Arterial
      line.
Disabled patient, abuse of, 2, 3
Discharge instructions, 89, 90i, 91-92
Discharge summary form, 90i
Distributive shock, 317t
DNR order. *See* Do-not-resuscitate
      order.
Doctor's orders clarification, 93
Documentation, correction to, 73
Do-not-resuscitate order, 94-95

Drug abuse, suspected, 154
Drug administration, 96, 97-98i
  one-time, 214-215
  stat order for, 321
Drug overdose, 99-100
Drug possession, illegal, 154-156
Drug refusal, 101
Drug search, conducting, 154-155
Duodenal feedings, 352-354
Durable power of attorney. *See*
      Advance directive.
Dyspnea, 102-104

E

Elder abuse, 2, 3
Elopement, 105
Emergency, informed consent and,
      165-166
Endotracheal extubation, 106-107
Endotracheal intubation, 108-109
Endotracheal tube removal by patient,
      110-111
Enema administration, 112-113
Epidural analgesia, 114-116
  adverse reactions to, 114
  flow sheet for, 115
Evidence collection, 117-119
  protocols for, 117

F

Fall precautions, 123-124
Falls, 120-122
  in acute care hospitals, 120
  in nursing homes, 120

Family questions about care, 127-128
Fluid deficit, 148-150
Foley catheter insertion, 358-359

G

Gastric lavage, 129-130
Gastrointestinal hemorrhage, 131-132
Glasgow Coma Scale, 186, 187i

H

Health Insurance Portability and
    Accountability Act, 133, 135
Heart attack, 204-206
Heat application, 136
Hemothorax, chest tube insertion
    for, 64
HIPAA. *See* Health Insurance
    Portability and Accountability
    Act.
Hyperglycemia, 137-138
Hypertensive crisis, 139-140
Hyperthermia-hypothermia blanket,
    141-142
Hypoglycemia, 143-144
Hypotension, 145-146
Hypovolemia, 148-150
Hypovolemic shock, 317t
Hypoxemia, 151-152

I

Illegal drug possession, 154-156
Implantable cardioverter-defibrillator,
    225

Incident report, 157-158, 159-160i
    tips for writing, 158
Incompetent patient, informed consent
    and, 163-164
Indwelling urinary catheter insertion,
    358-359
Infection control, 161-162
Infiltration, 178-179
Informed consent
    in emergency, 165-166
    inability to provide, 163-164
    for minor, 167
Intake and output, 168, 169i, 170
Intestinal obstruction, 171-172
I.V. catheter
    insertion of, 173-174
    removal of, 175
I.V. flow sheet, 180-181i
I.V. site
    caring for, 176
    change in, 177
    infiltration of, 178-179
    selection of, 173
I.V. therapy, 180-181

J

Jejunal feedings, 352-354
Joint Commission on Accreditation of
    Healthcare Organizations
    National Patient Safety Goals,
        386-391
    standards for restraint use, 309

i refers to an illustration; t refers to a table.

K
Katz index for activities of daily living assessment, 6

L
Large intestine, obstruction of, 171-172
Late documentation, 182
Late entries, 183
Latex hypersensitivity, 184-185
Lawton scale for activities of daily living assessment, 7
Level of consciousness, 186, 187i, 188
Levin tube. See Nasogastric tube.
Liability, reducing, in patient falls, 123
Life support termination, 189-190
Living will. See Advance directive.
Low blood pressure, 145-147
Lumbar puncture, 191-192

M
Mechanical ventilation, 193-194
Medical records, patient request to see, 240-241
Medication administration record, 96, 97-98i
Medication error, 195-196
    lawsuits and, 195
Medication event quality review form, 197-199i
Medication Kardex, 97-98i
Minor, informed consent for, 167
Missing patient, 105
Mistake on chart, correcting, 73
Moderate sedation, 200-201

Multiple trauma, 202-203
Myocardial infarction, 204-206

N
Nasogastric tube
    applications for, 209
    caring for patient with, 207
    insertion of, 209-210
    removal of, 211
Neglect, signs of, 3
Neurogenic shock, 317t
No-code order, 94-95
Noncompliance, 212
Nursing admission assessment, 12-14i
Nursing database, 11, 12-14i

O
One-time drug administration, 214-215
Operative site, marking, 338
Opioid control sheet, 217i
Opioid inventory, 216-217
    automated storage system and, 216
    government requirements for, 216
Order
    clarification of, 93
    do-not-resuscitate, 94-95
    no-code, 94-95
    stat drug administration, 321
    telephone, 344-345
    verbal, 360-361
    written, 372
Organ donation, 218-220
Ostomy care, 221-222
Oxygen administration, 223-224

P

Pacemaker
    malfunction of, 233-234
    permanent
        care of, 225-226
        insertion of, 227-228
    temporary, initiation of, 229-230
    transcutaneous, initiation of, 229-230
    transvenous, insertion of, 231-232
Pain flow sheet, 236i
Pain management, 235, 237
Pain scale, 236i
Patient, search of, 314-315
Patient authorization to use personal
        health information, 134i
Patient-controlled analgesia, 238
    flow sheet for, 239i
Patient falls, reducing liability in, 123
Patient request to see medical
        records, 240-241
Patient's belongings
    at admission, 242-243
    missing, 244-245
    search of, 314-315
Patient's bill of rights, 22
Patient self-glucose testing, 246-248
Patient teaching, 249, 254
    documenting, 255
    record of, 250-254i
Patient transfer
    to alternate care facility, 256,
        257-258i, 259-260
    to specialty unit, 261-262
Peripheral I.V. line. *See* I.V. catheter.

Peripherally inserted central catheter
    insertion of, 263-264
    site care for, 265-266
Peritoneal dialysis, 267-268
Peritoneal lavage, 269-270
Permanent pacemaker
    care of, 225-226
    insertion of, 227-228
Personal health information, patient
        authorization to use, 134i
Pneumonia, 271-272
Pneumothorax, 273-274
    chest tube insertion for, 64
Police custody of patient, 275-277
Postmortem care, 82-83
Postoperative care, 278-280
Postural drainage, 61
Preoperative care, 281, 282i
Preoperative surgical identification
        checklist, 340-341i
Preoperative verification process, 338
Pressure ulcer
    assessment of, 283, 288
        Braden scale for, 284-287t
    caring for, 289-290
Prisoner refusal of treatment, 276
Protected health information, 133
Pulmonary edema, 291-292
Pulse oximetry, 293-294

Q

Quality of care, family questions about,
        127-128

R

Rape trauma, 296-298

Rape-trauma syndrome, 296

Refusal of drugs, 101

Refusal of treatment, 299-301, 300i
  by prisoner, 276
  patient's right to, 299

Reportable communicable diseases,
  70-71

Reports to practitioner, 302-303

Respiratory arrest, 304-305

Respiratory distress, 306-308

Responsibility release form, 23i

Restraint use, 309, 312-313
  flow sheet for, 310-311i
  Joint Commission on Accreditation
    of Healthcare Organizations
    standards for, 309

Retention catheter insertion, 358-359

Risk assessment for falls, 125-126i

S

Safety device flow sheet, 310-311i

Salem sump tube. *See* Nasogastric
  tube.

Search and seizure laws, 118

Searches, guidelines for, 155

Search of patient or belongings,
  314-315

Sedation, moderate, 200-201

Self-glucose testing by patient, 246-248

Septic shock, 317t

Shock, 316, 318
  types of, 317t

Shortness of breath, 102-104

Side effect. *See* Adverse drug effects.

Single-dose drug administration,
  214-215

Skin care, 319-320

Small intestine, obstruction of, 171-172

Specialty unit, patient transfer to,
  261-262

Stat drug administration order, 321

Status asthmaticus, 322-324

Status epilepticus, 325-327

Stroke, 328-330

Substance withdrawal, 331-332

Suicidal patient, legal responsibilities
  when caring for, 333

Suicide precautions, 333-335

Surgical incision care, 336-337

Surgical site identification, 338-339, 341
  checklist for, 340-341i

Suture removal, 342-343

Synchronized cardioversion, 51-52

T

Telephone order, 344-345

Temporary pacemaker, initiation of,
  229-230

Thrombolytic therapy, 346-347

Tracheostomy
  caring for, 348-349
  suctioning, 350-351
  types of tubes for, 348

Transcultural assessment tool, 77-80i

Transcutaneous pacemaker initiation,
  229-230

Transfusion reaction report, 39i
Transvenous pacemaker insertion,
    231-232
Tube feeding, 352-354

U

Unlicensed assistive personnel care,
    355, 357
  supervising, 356
Urinary catheter (indwelling) insertion,
    358-359

V

Venipuncture device, selection of, 173
Ventilation, mechanical, 193-194
Verbal orders, 360-361
Visual analog pain scale, 236i
Vital signs, frequent, 362-363
  flow sheet for, 362-363i

WXYZ

Withholding an ordered medication,
    364-365, 365i
Wound assessment, 366, 367-368i, 369
Wound care, 370-371
Written orders, 372

i refers to an illustration; t refers to a table.

Notes

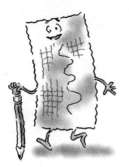

Notes

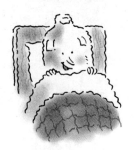

Notes

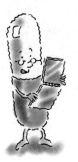